T0259281

Advances in the Diagnosis and Management of Barrett's Esophagus

Guest Editor

IRVING WAXMAN, MD, FASGE

GASTROINTESTINAL ENDOSCOPY CLINICS OF NORTH AMERICA

www.giendo.theclinics.com

Consulting Editor
CHARLES J. LIGHTDALE, MD

January 2011 • Volume 21 • Number 1

SAUNDERS an imprint of ELSEVIER, Inc.

W.B. SAUNDERS COMPANY
A Division of Elsevier Inc.

1600 John F. Kennedy Blvd. ● Suite 1800 ● Philadelphia, Pennsylvania 19103-2899

http://www.giendo.theclinics.com

GASTROINTESTINAL ENDOSCOPY CLINICS OF NORTH AMERICA Volume 21, Number 1
January 2011 ISSN 1052-5157, ISBN-13: 978-1-4557-0452-1

Editor: Kerry Holland
Developmental Editor: Donald Mumford

Gastrointestinal Endoscopy Clinics of North America (ISSN 1052-5157) is published quarterly by Elsevier Inc., 360 Park Avenue South, New York, NY 10010-1710. Months of issue are January, April, July, and October. Business and Editorial Offices: 1600 John F. Kennedy Blvd., Suite 1800, Philadelphia, PA, 19103-2899. Periodicals postage paid at New York, NY and additional mailing offices. Subscription prices are $295.00 per year for US individuals, $414.00 per year for US institutions, $156.00 per year for US students and residents, $325.00 per year for Canadian individuals, $505.00 per year for Canadian institutions, $412.00 per year for international individuals, $505.00 per year for international institutions, and $217.00 per year for Canadian and foreign students/residents. To receive student/resident rate, orders must be accompanied by name of affiliated institution, date of term, and the *signature* of program/residency coordinator on institution letterhead. Orders will be billed at individual rate until proof of status is received. Foreign air speed delivery is included in all *Clinics* subscription prices. All prices are subject to change without notice. **POSTMASTER:** Send address change to *Gastrointestinal Endoscopy Clinics of North America*, Elsevier Health Sciences Division, Subscription Customer Service, 3251 Riverport Lane, Maryland Heights, MO 63043. **Customer Service: 1-800-654-2452 (US). From outside the United States, call 1-314-447-8871. Fax: 1-314-447-8029. E-mail: JournalsCustomerService-usa@elsevier.com (for print support) or JournalsOnlineSupport-usa@elsevier.com (for online support).**

Reprints. For copies of 100 or more, of articles in this publication, please contact the Commercial Reprints Department, Elsevier Inc., 360 Park Avenue South, New York, NY 10010-1710. Tel. (212) 633-3812; Fax: (212) 482-1935; E-mail: reprints@elsevier.com.

Gastrointestinal Endoscopy Clinics of North America is covered in *Excerpta Medica, MEDLINE/PubMed (Index Medicus),* and *MEDLINE/MEDLARS.*

Printed and bound by CPI Group (UK) Ltd, Croydon, CR0 4YY

Transferred to Digital Print 2011

Contributors

CONSULTING EDITOR

CHARLES J. LIGHTDALE, MD
Professor, Department of Medicine, Columbia University Medical Center, New York, New York

GUEST EDITOR

IRVING WAXMAN, MD, FASGE
Professor of Medicine and Surgery, Director, Center for Endoscopic Research and Therapeutics (CERT), Section of Gastroenterology, Department of Medicine, The University of Chicago Medical Center, Chicago, Illinois

AUTHORS

WILLIAM J. BULSIEWICZ, MD, MSc
Fellow, GI Outcomes Training Program, Division of Gastroenterology, University of North Carolina School of Medicine, Chapel Hill, North Carolina

NAVTEJ S. BUTTAR, MD
Assistant Professor of Medicine, Division of Gastroenterology, Mayo Clinic, Rochester, Minnesota

ANN M. CHEN, MD
Director of Endoscopic Ultrasound, Assistant Professor, Division of Gastroenterology and Hepatology, Stanford University School of Medicine, Stanford University Medical Center, Redwood City, California

JENNIFER CHENNAT, MD
Assistant Professor of Medicine, Section of Gastroenterology, Department of Medicine, Center for Endoscopic Research and Therapeutics (CERT), The University of Chicago Medical Center, Chicago, Illinois

MARTA L. DAVILA, MD
Professor of Medicine, Department of Gastroenterology, Hepatology and Nutrition, The University of Texas MD Anderson Cancer Center, Houston, Texas

CHRISTIAN ELL, MD, PhD
Professor of Medicine, Head of the Department of Internal Medicine 2, HSK Wiesbaden, Wiesbaden, Germany

GARY W. FALK, MD, MS
Professor of Medicine, Division of Gastroenterology, Department of Internal Medicine, Hospital of the University of Pennsylvania, Philadelphia, Pennsylvania

MARK K. FERGUSON, MD
Professor of Surgery, Section of Thoracic Surgery, Department of Surgery, The University of Chicago Medical Center, Chicago, Illinois

FERNANDO A.M. HERBELLA, MD
Research Associate, Department of Surgery, University of Chicago Pritzker School of Medicine, Chicago, Illinois

PATRICIA A. HOOPER, MBChB(Leics), BSc(Leics)
Digestive Diseases Centre, Leicester Royal Infirmary, Leicester, United Kingdom

JANUSZ A. JANKOWSKI, MSc(Oxon), MD(Dund), PhD(Lond), FRCP(Lond), FACG(USA)
Digestive Diseases Centre, Leicester Royal Infirmary, Leicester; Department of Clinical Pharmacology, University of Oxford, Oxford; Centre for Digestive Diseases, Queen Mary University of London, London, United Kingdom

BRYSON W. KATONA, MD, PhD
Department of Internal Medicine, Hospital of the University of Pennsylvania, Philadelphia, Pennsylvania

VANI J.A. KONDA, MD
Instructor of Medicine, Section of Gastroenterology, Department of Medicine, The University of Chicago Medical Center, Chicago, Illinois

ALBERTO LARGHI, MD, PhD
Digestive Endoscopy Unit, Universita' Cattolica del Sacro Cuore, Rome, Italy

HENDRIK MANNER, MD, PhD
Department of Internal Medicine 2, HSK Wiesbaden, Wiesbaden, Germany

V. RAMAN MUTHUSAMY, MD
Associate Clinical Professor of Medicine and Fellowship Director, Division of Gastroenterology, University of California, Irvine, Orange, California

NGOZI OKORO, MD
Division of Gastroenterology, Mayo Clinic, Rochester, Minnesota

PANKAJ J. PASRICHA, MD
Professor and Chief, Division of Gastroenterology and Hepatology, Stanford University School of Medicine, Stanford University Medical Center, Stanford, California

MARCO G. PATTI, MD
Professor of Surgery and Director of the Center for Esophageal Diseases, Department of Surgery, University of Chicago Pritzker School of Medicine, Chicago, Illinois

OLIVER PECH, MD, PhD
Co-Director of the Endoscopy Unit, Department of Internal Medicine 2, HSK Wiesbaden, Wiesbaden, Germany

GANAPATHY PRASAD, MD
Assistant Professor of Medicine, Division of Gastroenterology, Mayo Clinic, Rochester, Minnesota

TOM C.J. SEERDEN, MD, PhD
Departement of Gastroenterology, Amphia Hospital, Breda, The Netherlands

NICHOLAS J. SHAHEEN, MD, MPH
Professor of Medicine and Epidemiology, Director, Center for Esophageal Diseases and Swallowing, Division of Gastroenterology, University of North Carolina School of Medicine, Chapel Hill, North Carolina

PRATEEK SHARMA, MD
Professor of Medicine and Fellowship Director, Division of Gastroenterology, Department of Medicine, University of Kansas Medical Center, Kansas City, Kansas; Veterans Administration Medical Center, Kansas City, Missouri

RHONDA F. SOUZA, MD
Associate Professor, Department of Medicine, Veterans Affairs North Texas Health Care System and the University of Texas Southwestern Medical School; Department of Medicine, Harold C. Simmons Comprehensive Cancer Center, University of Texas Southwestern Medical Center at Dallas, Dallas, Texas

STUART JON SPECHLER, MD
Department of Medicine, Veterans Affairs North Texas Healthcare System; Professor of Medicine, Berta M. and Cecil O. Patterson Chair in Gastroenterology, University of Texas Southwestern Medical Center; Chief, Division of Gastroenterology, Dallas Veterans Affairs Medical Center, Dallas, Texas

JIANMIN TIAN, MD
Division of Gastroenterology, Mayo Clinic, Rochester, Minnesota

DAVID H. WANG, MD, PhD
Assistant Professor, Department of Medicine, Veterans Affairs North Texas Health Care System and the University of Texas Southwestern Medical School; Department of Medicine, Harold C. Simmons Comprehensive Cancer Center, University of Texas Southwestern Medical Center at Dallas; Division of Hematology-Oncology (111C), Dallas Veterans Affairs Medical Center, Dallas, Texas

KENNETH K. WANG, MD
Professor of Medicine, Division of Gastroenterology, Mayo Clinic, Rochester, Minnesota

IRVING WAXMAN, MD, FASGE
Professor of Medicine and Surgery, Director, Center for Endoscopic Research and Therapeutics (CERT), Section of Gastroenterology, Department of Medicine, The University of Chicago Medical Center, Chicago, Illinois

MICHEL WONGKEESONG, MD
Assistant Professor of Medicine, Division of Gastroenterology, Mayo Clinic, Rochester, Minnesota

Contents

Barrett's esophagus has been defined conceptually as the condition in which any extent of metaplastic columnar epithelium that predisposes to cancer development replaces the stratified squamous epithelium that normally lines the distal esophagus. The condition develops as a consequence of gastroesophageal reflux disease. Barrett's metaplasia has clinical importance primarily because of its malignant predisposition, and virtually all of the contentious clinical issues in Barrett's esophagus are related in some way to its cancer risk. This article considers some key clinical issues that impact the management of patients with Barrett's esophagus.

Barrett's esophagus is a well-known risk factor for the development of esophageal adenocarcinoma. Current practice guidelines recommend endoscopic surveillance of patients with Barrett's esophagus in an attempt to detect cancer at an early and potentially curable stage. This review addresses the rationale behind surveillance and criteria for inclusion of patients in surveillance programs as well as the appropriate technique and intervals that should be used. This work addresses other key topics in Barrett's esophagus surveillance, including the efficacy of surveillance programs, physician compliance with surveillance guidelines, cost-effectiveness of surveillance programs, and areas for future research.

The past few years have brought new advances in our understanding of the molecular mechanisms underlying the development of Barrett's esophagus and esophageal adenocarcinoma. Although knowledge of the genetic basis for these conditions has not yet translated into clinically useful biomarkers, the current pace of biomedical discovery holds endless possibilities for molecular medicine to improve the diagnosis and management of patients with these conditions. This article provides a useful conceptual basis for understanding the molecular events involved in the making of Barrett metaplasia and in its neoplastic progression, and provides a rationale for evaluating studies on the application of molecular medicine to the diagnosis and management of patients with Barrett's esophagus and esophageal adenocarcinoma.

Enhanced visualization techniques are available for Barrett's esophagus and have promise in the detection of dysplasia and cancer. Several of these techniques, such as narrow band imaging and chromoendoscopy, are being applied clinically. These techniques will allow the endoscopist to screen the surface of the Barrett's esophagus to detect areas of neoplasia. Once detected, it is hoped that either magnification techniques, such as confocal laser endomicroscopy, or spectroscopic techniques can be of value in allowing in vivo real-time diagnostic capabilities.

The main goal in the staging of patients with early neoplasia arising in the context of Barrett's esophagus (BE) is to identify individuals who are eligible for endoscopic therapy and differentiate them from those who require surgical management. To make the proper patient selection a combined staging strategy consisting of endoscopy evaluation, endoscopic ultrasonography, and endoscopic mucosal resection is necessary. In this article, the authors summarize the evidence behind each different staging modality in the setting of early BE adenocarcinoma and propose a staging approach that helps to select patients who are suitable for endoscopic therapy.

Photodynamic therapy (PDT) is a photochemical process that uses a photosensitizer drug activated by laser light to produce mucosal ablation. Porfimer sodium PDT has proved long-term efficacy and durability in the treatment of Barrett's esophagus and high-grade dysplasia and early esophageal adenocarcinoma. Its use has been limited by serious side effects including prolonged cutaneous photosensitivity and stricture formation. Other photosensitizers with a better safety profile have been used mostly in Europe with limited experience. The future of PDT lies on a better understanding of dosimetry, tissue properties, and host genetic factors.

Endoscopic resection (ER) has become the most important endoscopic treatment method of early cancers of the upper GI tract. ER serves as a therapeutic but also as a diagnostic tool by providing a specimen for histologic assessment. In expert hands ER is easy to performa and has a very low complication rate. Long-term results in early esophageal and gastric cancer are excellent.

Studies in the last several years have consistently shown radiofrequency ablation (RFA) to be effective, safe, and well tolerated in the treatment of

nondysplastic and dysplastic Barrett's esophagus (BE). The results found at
academic medical centers have been reproduced in the community setting.
RFA provides a safe and cost-effective alternative to surgery or surveillance
in the management of high-grade dysplasia (HGD). RFA should be given
serious consideration as first-line therapy for HGD. This article reviews
the evidence behind RFA to differentiate it from other management
strategies in terms of efficacy, durability, safety, tolerability, and cost-
effectiveness. The role of RFA in the management of BE is described,
including endoscopic resection. Future directions are identified for research
that will help to better define the role of RFA in the management of BE.

Cryotherapy is a noncontact ablation method that has long been used clinically in the treatment of a wide variety of malignant and premalignant diseases. The relative ease of use and unique mechanisms of cellular
destruction make cryotherapy particularly attractive for the eradication
of dysplastic Barrett's esophagus. Currently, liquid nitrogen and carbon
dioxide are the most common cryogens used. Preliminary data with these
agents have shown high efficacy in the reversal of dysplastic Barrett
mucosa and excellent safety profiles. Intense investigation on cryotherapy
ablation of Barrett's esophagus is ongoing.

Recent developments in endoscopic therapeutic options for Barrett's
esophagus (BE) early neoplasia have resulted in a dramatic paradigm shift
in its clinical management. With multiple endoscopic choices available, it is
important to discern subtle differences between these approaches based
on the available current data and known limitations of each modality. The
goals of endoscopic therapy of Barrett's neoplasia are to preserve the
esophagus while ablating or removing the entire BE segment. This article
reviews the currently available BE endoscopic treatments with emphasis
on appropriate selection of patients, indications and timing of use, and
clinical management considerations.

Gastroesophageal reflux disease (GERD) is a highly prevalent disease.
Population studies have demonstrated that a significant proportion of individuals weekly experience GERD symptoms. Barrett's esophagus (BE),
defined by the presence of intestinal metaplasia (columnar epithelium
with goblet cells), is considered a consequence of chronic reflux. This
review defines the role of surgery in the modern treatment of BE, taking
into consideration the pathophysiology of the disease and the new endoscopic procedures available at present.

Advances in the development of endoscopic therapies for Barrett's esophagus have resulted in the emergence of an important paradigm shift for

management of early neoplasia and represent an opportunity to alter the natural history of the disease. Clinical incorporation of these endoscopic modalities may have significant implications for disease management and health care delivery from a cost perspective. This article reviews the current literature on the cost analyses of commonly used Barrett endoscopic interventions and summarizes the overall cost-effectiveness of these treatments as compared with surveillance or surgery.

Esophageal adenocarcinoma is increasing in incidence. The main risk factor is the premalignant condition of Barrett's esophagus. There is great interest in chemoprevention to prevent or slow malignant transformation. There are many agents proposed as playing a role in chemoprevention; however, none is licensed for this role as yet. Aspirin possesses many favorable qualities for chemoprevention and is the focus of the largest randomized control trial in this field.

The past decade has led to marked improvements in our understanding regarding the pathogenesis and risk of progression of Barrett's esophagus (BE), enhanced imaging technology to improve dysplasia detection, and the development and refinement of endoscopic techniques, such as mucosal ablation and endoscopic mucosal resection(EMR), to eradicate BE. However, many questions remain including identifying which, if any, candidates are most appropriate for screening for BE; how to improve current surveillance protocols; predicting which patients with BE will develop neoplastic progression; identifying the most appropriate candidates for endoscopic eradication therapy; developing algorithms for appropriate management posteradication; and understanding the potential role of chemoprophylaxis. This article describes potential future advances regarding screening, surveillance, risk stratification, endoscopic eradication therapies, and chemoprevention and provides a potential future management strategy for patients with BE.

RELATED INTEREST

Gastroenterology Clinics of North America, December 2010 (Vol. 39, No. 4)
Advanced Imaging in Gastroenterology
Ralf Kiesslich, MD, *Guest Editor*

THE CLINICS ARE NOW AVAILABLE ONLINE!

Access your subscription at:
www.theclinics.com

Foreword

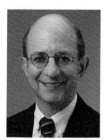

Charles J. Lightdale, MD
Consulting Editor

The continuing dramatic rise in the incidence of esophageal adenocarcinoma has driven progress in our understanding and management of Barrett's esophagus, the premalignant condition most associated with this highly lethal cancer. The relatively easy accessibility of Barrett's esophagus to the gastrointestinal endoscopist has also resulted in new approaches in prevention, early detection, and treatment. Exciting new discoveries in understanding carcinogenesis in Barrett's tissue have emerged, along with new optical methods for identification of early neoplasia in Barrett's epithelium. Progress has been most notable in the endoscopic treatment of early neoplasia in Barrett's esophagus, where endoscopic mucosal resection and radiofrequency ablation have become important and demonstrably effective new approaches. Dr Irving Waxman, the guest editor for this issue of *Gastrointestinal Endoscopy Clinics of North America,* is one of the foremost leaders in this field. He has gathered an international group of experts to document the progress, to update new technologies and insights that can be applied now, and to open a window into the future.

Charles J. Lightdale, MD
Department of Medicine
Columbia University Medical Center
161 Fort Washington Avenue, Room 812
New York, NY 10032, USA

E-mail address:
CJL18@columbia.edu

Gastrointest Endoscopy Clin N Am 21 (2011) xiii
doi:10.1016/j.giec.2010.10.003
1052-5157/11/$ — see front matter © 2011 Elsevier Inc. All rights reserved.

giendo.theclinics.com

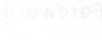

Preface

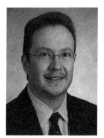

Irving Waxman, MD
Guest Editor

Barrett's esophagus (BE) is clearly recognized as the most important risk factor for the development of esophageal adenocarcinoma. The incidence of this cancer has increased by approximately sixfold during the last 30 years, a rate greater than that of any other cancer in the United States during this period of time. Matching this challenge, the past decade has seen marked advances in our understanding of the risk of neoplastic progression in BE, new and promising endoscopic imaging technologies for identification of dysplasia, and the development of numerous modalities to achieve endoscopic eradiation of this tissue. Nevertheless, the answers today to the fundamental questions of in whom, when, how, and which techniques to perform screening, surveillance, and treatment remain elusive. The goal of this issue of the *Gastrointestinal Endoscopy Clinics of North America* is to provide the clinician up-to-date information on what is known today in the evaluation and management of BE and to discuss the unmet needs in understanding the biology of the disease as well as strategies for intervention ranging from chemoprevention to ablative technologies and ultimately the role of surgery. We are fortunate to have an internationally recognized cadre of experts in the field discussing all clinical and controversial aspects of the disease and providing a balanced opinion regarding its evaluation and management.

We also have asked our experts to give us a glimpse into the future and predict what breakthroughs the next decade will bring in cost-effective screening and surveillance, risk stratification, and tailored interventions based on risk for development of esophageal adenocarcinoma.

I want to express my sincere thanks to Dr Charles Lightdale, Consulting Editor, for allowing me the opportunity to put together this exciting issue as well as to a wonderful group of talented and expert opinion leaders who kindly agreed to share their time and knowledge to this project.

I hope our readers will find this issue useful when managing patients with BE as well as to challenge investigators in the field to find the answers to some of the many questions raised in this volume.

Gastrointest Endoscopy Clin N Am 21 (2011) xv–xvi
doi:10.1016/j.giec.2010.10.002
1052-5157/11/$ – see front matter

In the words of the French author Andre Gide, *"Man cannot discover new oceans unless he has the courage to lose sight of the shore."*

Irving Waxman, MD
Center for Endoscopic Research and Therapeutics (CERT)
The University of Chicago
5758 South Maryland Avenue, MC 9028
Chicago, IL 60637-1463, USA

E-mail address:
iwaxman@uchicago.edu

Barrett's Esophagus: Clinical Issues

Stuart Jon Spechler, MD[a,b,c],*

KEYWORDS

- Barrett's esophagus • Gastroesophageal reflux disease
- Intestinal metaplasia • Esophageal adenocarcinoma

Barrett's esophagus has been defined conceptually as the condition in which any extent of metaplastic columnar epithelium that predisposes to cancer development replaces the stratified squamous epithelium that normally lines the distal esophagus.[1] The condition develops as a consequence of gastroesophageal reflux disease (GERD). Barrett's metaplasia has clinical importance primarily because of its malignant predisposition, and virtually all of the contentious clinical issues in Barrett's esophagus are related in some way to its cancer risk. This article considers some key clinical issues that impact the management of patients with Barrett's esophagus.

DIAGNOSIS

Although more than 60 years have passed since Barrett[2] published his original treatise on the condition that now bears his name, authorities still dispute the diagnostic criteria for Barrett's esophagus. The conceptual definition proposed in the introduction does not translate readily into clear-cut diagnostic criteria, in part because it is not clear which of the multiple columnar cell types that can be found in Barrett's esophagus have a malignant predisposition.

In 1976, Paull and colleagues[3] reported that patients with Barrett's esophagus could have up to three types of columnar epithelia lining the distal esophagus: (1) a junctional (also called "cardia-type") epithelium comprised of mucus-secreting cells; (2) a gastric fundic-type epithelium with parietal and chief cells; and (3) intestinal-type metaplasia (also called "specialized columnar epithelium" or "specialized intestinal metaplasia") with prominent goblet cells. By the early 1980s, it had been established that Barrett's esophagus was a risk factor for esophageal adenocarcinoma, and intestinal metaplasia was reported to be the esophageal epithelial type

Supported by the Office of Medical Research, Department of Veterans Affairs and the National Institutes of Health (DK63621 to R.F.S.)

[a] Department of Medicine, Veterans Affairs North Texas Healthcare System, Dallas, TX, USA
[b] University of Texas Southwestern Medical Center, Dallas, TX 75216, USA
[c] Division of Gastroenterology, Dallas Veterans Affairs Medical Center, 4500 South Lancaster Road, Dallas, TX 75216, USA
* Corresponding author. University of Texas Southwestern Medical Center, Dallas, TX 75216.
E-mail address: SJSpechler@AOL.com

Gastrointest Endoscopy Clin N Am 21 (2011) 1–7
doi:10.1016/j.giec.2010.09.012
1052-5157/11/$ – see front matter. Published by Elsevier Inc.

giendo.theclinics.com

most frequently associated with that cancer.[4] By the late 1980s, intestinal metaplasia was widely regarded as both the most common type of Barrett's epithelium and the one that predisposed to malignancy.[5] In addition, intestinal metaplasia was readily identified histologically by its distinctive goblet cells and, unlike the cardia-type and gastric fundic-type epithelia, intestinal metaplasia clearly was abnormal when found in the region of the gastroesophageal junction. Consequently, some authorities chose to define Barrett's esophagus by the presence of intestinal metaplasia, and this diagnostic criterion was adopted into clinical practice.[5] Since the 1990s, an esophageal biopsy specimen showing intestinal-type metaplasia with goblet cells has become virtually a sine qua non for the diagnosis of Barrett's esophagus.[6]

In 1994, Spechler and colleagues[7] reported that 18% of consecutive patients in a general endoscopy unit who had columnar epithelium that involved less than 3 cm of the distal esophagus had intestinal metaplasia. Before then, endoscopists infrequently took biopsy specimens from such short segments of esophageal columnar epithelium. Since then, Barrett's esophagus has been categorized as long-segment (when the metaplastic epithelium extends ≥3 cm above the gastroesophageal junction) or short-segment (when there is <3 cm of metaplastic epithelium lining the esophagus).[8] The Prague C and M classification, which calls for identifying both the circumferential extent (C) and the maximum extent (M) of Barrett's metaplasia, is an even more recent system for describing the extent of Barrett's esophagus endoscopically.[9] Although studies have demonstrated excellent interobserver agreement among endoscopists using the Prague C and M criteria (when columnar epithelium extends >1 cm above the gastroesophageal junction), the clinical benefit of using this system has not been established and, presently, patients with any extent of intestinal metaplasia in the esophagus are managed similarly.

When evaluating studies on Barrett's esophagus, physicians should consider how changes in diagnostic criteria over the years have impacted the conclusions of those investigations. For example, short-segment Barrett's esophagus was not widely recognized until 1994, and most studies reported before that year included only patients with long-segment disease. More recent studies, however, include a substantial proportion of short-segment Barrett's patients whose GERD severity and esophageal cancer risk may differ considerably from those for patients with long-segment disease. It may not be appropriate to extrapolate the results of older studies on the epidemiology and natural history of long-segment Barrett's esophagus to patients with short-segment disease.

Another recent issue that has caused considerable controversy is whether the diagnosis of Barrett's esophagus should be limited to patients who have an esophageal biopsy specimen demonstrating intestinal metaplasia (with goblet cells), or whether the finding of gastric cardia-type epithelium in the esophagus also warrants that diagnosis.[10] Cardia-type epithelium traditionally has been considered the normal lining of the proximal stomach (the gastric cardia). However, there are data to suggest that cardia-type epithelium might not be normal, but rather a metaplastic lining that develops as a consequence of GERD.[11] Histochemical and molecular studies of cardia-type epithelium have revealed abnormalities that could predispose to carcinogenesis,[12,13] and several limited clinical studies support the concept that cardia-type epithelium has malignant potential.[14–16] Consequently, some authorities have proposed that cardia-type epithelium in the esophagus should be considered Barrett's esophagus.[10]

Most studies of cancer risk in Barrett's esophagus have included patients with intestinal metaplasia, either primarily or exclusively. Therefore, the magnitude of the cancer risk associated with cardia-type epithelium in the esophagus is not clear.

Pending such clarification, it seems reasonable to limit the diagnosis of Barrett's esophagus to patients who have intestinal metaplasia. This diagnostic criterion could change in the near future. However, it should be noted that the conceptual definition of Barrett's esophagus (the condition in which any extent of metaplastic columnar epithelium that predisposes to cancer development replaces the stratified squamous epithelium that normally lines the distal esophagus) does not change, even if specific diagnostic criteria are altered.

PREVALENCE

Barrett's esophagus (predominantly the short-segment variety) is found in 10% to 20% of patients who have endoscopic examinations for the evaluation of GERD symptoms.[17] Two relatively recent studies have provided information on the prevalence of Barrett's esophagus in the general population.[18,19] In one study from Sweden, 1000 randomly selected adults in the general population had an endoscopic examination performed to look for Barrett's esophagus.[18] The condition was identified endoscopically and confirmed by an esophageal biopsy specimen showing intestinal metaplasia in 16 individuals (5 long- and 11 short-segment Barrett's esophagus), representing an overall prevalence of 1.6%. This prevalence rate is likely an underestimate, however, because 60 patients (6%) were found to have intestinal metaplasia in biopsy specimens taken at the gastroesophageal junction, and some of those patients probably had short-segment Barrett's esophagus that was not recognized by the endoscopists. Interestingly, only 9 (56%) of the 16 individuals identified with Barrett's esophagus had a history of GERD symptoms (4 [80%] of the 5 with long- and 5 of [46%] of the 11 with short-segment Barrett's esophagus). In an American study in which 961 patients scheduled for elective colonoscopy agreed to have an upper gastrointestinal endoscopy performed to detect Barrett's esophagus, the overall prevalence of the condition was 6.8%.[19] Among the 556 patients who had no history of heartburn, short-segment Barrett's esophagus was found in 5.2%, whereas 5.7% of 384 patients who complained of heartburn had short-segment Barrett's esophagus.

The aforementioned studies suggest that the prevalence of Barrett's esophagus in the general adult population is between 2% and 7%. Clearly, Barrett's esophagus is a very common condition. The studies also suggest that GERD is not a reliable marker for Barrett's esophagus, especially the short-segment variety. These observations have at least two important implications for clinicians who treat patients with Barrett's esophagus. First, because the condition is so common, virtually any interventional management strategy applied to the general population of patients with Barrett's esophagus entails a considerable health care expenditure for society. Second, screening programs for the condition that include only patients with GERD symptoms miss approximately 50% of individuals who have Barrett's esophagus.

CANCER RISK

Published estimates on the incidence of cancer in Barrett's esophagus have ranged from 0.2% to 2.9% per year.[20] By pooling data from those reports, investigators in the 1990s estimated that patients with Barrett's esophagus developed cancer at the rate of 1% per year.[21] In 2000, Shaheen and colleagues[20] reported that this estimate was too high, because many of the studies on which the estimate was based were small series, and those reports suffered from publication bias (the selective reporting of studies with positive or extreme results). Presently, the risk of cancer in Barrett's esophagus is judged to be approximately 0.5% per year.

Although the difference between an annual cancer incidence of 0.5% and 1% may seem trivial, this difference has important implications for the management of patients with Barrett's esophagus. Computer models on the value of different endoscopic surveillance and interventional strategies for patients with Barrett's esophagus can be extremely sensitive to the value chosen for the incidence of esophageal cancer. In one such model, for example, endoscopic surveillance every 2 years is the preferred strategy if the annual cancer incidence is 1%, whereas surveillance every 4 years is preferred for an annual cancer incidence of 0.5%.[22]

One important consideration when evaluating reports on the risk of cancer in Barrett's esophagus is the year of publication. As already discussed, short-segment Barrett's esophagus was not widely recognized before 1994, and reports published before then included patients with long-segment disease exclusively. It is logical to assume that the risk of cancer in Barrett's esophagus should increase with the extent of metaplastic epithelium. Patients with longer segments of metaplasia have more cells at risk for mutation and, therefore, should be more likely to acquire the critical combination of DNA alterations that results in malignancy. Data from a number of observational studies support this hypothesis,[23–25] but there is no proof that the risk of cancer in Barrett's esophagus varies with the extent of the metaplastic lining.[26]

Some very recent studies have described rates of cancer development in Barrett's esophagus considerably lower than the widely accepted estimate of 0.5% per year. In a cohort of 1203 patients with Barrett's esophagus from five different medical centers who were followed for a mean duration of 5.5 years (6644 patient-years), for example, Wani and colleagues[27] found that only 18 patients developed esophageal adenocarcinoma, which represents a cancer incidence rate of only 0.27% per year (0.17%–0.43%, 95% confidence interval). Indeed, 99% of the 504 patients who were followed for 5 years remained cancer-free. It is not clear whether this surprisingly low rate of cancer development was caused by the inclusion of a large number of patients with short-segment Barrett's esophagus, the result of aggressive acid-suppressive therapy, or caused by other, unknown factors.

DOES THE CANCER RISK JUSTIFY INVASIVE THERAPY FOR PATIENTS WITH NONDYSPLASTIC BARRETT'S ESOPHAGUS?

For reasons that are not well understood, the frequency of esophageal adenocarcinoma has increased profoundly in the United States over the past several decades.[28] Barrett's esophagus is a major risk factor for this lethal tumor, and a number of invasive therapies (discussed elsewhere in this issue) are available to eradicate Barrett's metaplasia. As discussed, however, the risk of developing esophageal adenocarcinoma for individual patients who have Barrett's esophagus (without dysplasia) is low. This low rate of cancer progression raises concerns regarding the invasive treatment options. Does the benefit of an invasive procedure in preventing esophageal cancer justify the expense, inconvenience, and risks of the procedure for patients who have Barrett's esophagus without dysplasia?

A recent randomized, sham-controlled trial of radiofrequency ablation (RFA) for patients with high-grade dysplasia in Barrett's esophagus has demonstrated that RFA, which has few serious side effects, decreases the progression from high-grade dysplasia to cancer at 1 year.[29] Limited, uncontrolled studies also have shown that RFA can eradicate nondysplastic Barrett's epithelium safely in most patients.[30] Noting these results, some authorities recently have proposed that RFA should be considered a therapeutic option to prevent cancer for patients who have Barrett's esophagus without dysplasia.[31] Their arguments are summarized next. (1) Nondysplastic Barrett's metaplasia frequently shows clonal molecular abnormalities that might predispose to cancer development. (2) The common clinical practice of performing endoscopic surveillance to detect curable neoplasia for patients with Barrett's esophagus is of limited benefit because dysplasia and cancer can be missed as a result of endoscopic biopsy sampling error; the interpretation of dysplasia by pathologists is subjective and inconsistent; patient and physician compliance with surveillance guidelines can be poor; and even with perfect compliance, cancers in Barrett's esophagus have developed without apparent antecedent dysplasia. (3) RFA safely eliminates Barrett's metaplasia in most cases and the results seem to be durable for up to 5 years in limited series. So, why not be proactive and ablate Barrett's metaplasia with RFA rather than relying on endoscopic surveillance, which has dubious efficacy?

The counterarguments to the proposal for RFA treatment of nondysplastic Barrett's esophagus are as follows. (1) Despite the molecular abnormalities that can be found in nondysplastic Barrett's metaplasia, the rate of cancer development is low and adenocarcinoma of the esophagus remains an uncommon malignancy in the general population. (2) RFA may be safe compared with esophagectomy or with photodynamic therapy, but RFA has complications including esophageal stricture formation and bleeding. (3) RFA is a relatively new procedure and long-term results simply are not available. Although the results of RFA seem to be durable in very limited data extending to 5 years, the frequency of "buried metaplasia" (Barrett's metaplasia concealed by an overlying layer of squamous epithelium following ablation) and the long-term frequency of recurrent metaplasia are not known. (4) There are no data showing that RFA prevents cancer for patients with nondysplastic Barrett's metaplasia. (5) In the absence of long-term data on the rate of recurrent metaplasia and efficacy in cancer prevention, patients who have had RFA will likely require continued endoscopic surveillance, with its attendant expense and inconvenience. (6) RFA is expensive. Using a combination of circumferential and focal RFA procedures, one uncontrolled study found complete eradication of Barrett's epithelium in 60 (98%) of 61 patients.[30] However, this required a mean of 1.5 circumferential ablations and 1.9 focal ablations for each patient, representing considerable expense.

SUMMARY

The prevalence of Barrett's esophagus in the general adult population is between 2% and 7%. For such a common condition, interventional management strategies entail a considerable health care expenditure for society. When used in so many patients, furthermore, even a relatively safe procedure as RFA results in a substantial number of complications. Does the potential, but unproved, benefit of RFA in preventing cancer justify the enormous expense (three to four RFA procedures per patient to eliminate Barrett's metaplasia), inconvenience, and risk of a procedure that presently does not even eliminate the need for regular endoscopic surveillance?

REFERENCES

1. Spechler SJ, Fitzgerald RC, Prasad GA, et al. History, molecular mechanisms, and endoscopic treatment of Barrett's esophagus. Gastroenterology 2010;138: 854–69.
2. Barrett NR. Chronic peptic ulcer of the oesophagus and "oesophagitis." Br J Surg 1950;38:175–82.
3. Paull A, Trier JS, Dalton MD, et al. The histologic spectrum of Barrett's esophagus. N Engl J Med 1976;295:476–80.

4. Haggitt RC, Dean PJ. Adenocarcinoma in Barrett's epithelium. In: Spechler SJ, Goyal RK, editors. Barrett's esophagus: pathophysiology, diagnosis, and management. New York: Elsevier Science Publishing; 1985. p. 153–66.

5. Reid BJ. Barrett's esophagus and esophageal adenocarcinoma. Gastroenterol Clin North Am 1991;20:817–34.

6. Weinstein WM, Ippoliti AF. The diagnosis of Barrett's esophagus: goblets, goblets, goblets. Gastrointest Endosc 1996;44:91–5.

7. Spechler SJ, Zeroogian JM, Antonioli DA, et al. Prevalence of metaplasia at the gastro-oesophageal junction. Lancet 1994;344:1533–6.

8. Sharma P, Morales TG, Sampliner RE. Short segment Barrett's esophagus. The need for standardization of the definition and of endoscopic criteria. Am J Gastroenterol 1998;93:1033–6.

9. Sharma P, Dent J, Armstrong D, et al. The development and validation of an endoscopic grading system for Barrett's esophagus: the Prague C & M criteria. Gastroenterology 2006;131:1392–9.

10. Riddell RH, Odze RD. Definition of Barrett's esophagus: time for a rethink–is intestinal metaplasia dead? Am J Gastroenterol 2009;104:2588–94.

11. Chandrasoma P. Pathophysiology of Barrett's esophagus. Semin Thorac Cardiovasc Surg 1997;9:270–8.

12. Liu W, Hahn H, Odze RD, et al. Metaplastic esophageal columnar epithelium without goblet cells shows DNA content abnormalities similar to goblet cell-containing epithelium. Am J Gastroenterol 2009;104:816–24.

13. Hahn HP, Blount PL, Ayub K, et al. Intestinal differentiation in metaplastic, non-goblet columnar epithelium in the esophagus. Am J Surg Pathol 2009;33:1006–15.

14. Takubo K, Aida J, Naomoto Y, et al. Cardiac rather than intestinal-type background in endoscopic resection specimens of minute Barrett adenocarcinoma. Hum Pathol 2009;40:65–74.

15. Kelty CJ, Gough MD, Van Wyk Q, et al. Barrett's oesophagus: intestinal metaplasia is not essential for cancer risk. Scand J Gastroenterol 2007;42:1271–4.

16. Gatenby PA, Ramus JR, Caygill CP, et al. Relevance of the detection of intestinal metaplasia in non-dysplastic columnar-lined oesophagus. Scand J Gastroenterol 2008;43:524–30.

17. Spechler SJ. Barrett's esophagus. N Engl J Med 2002;346:836–42.

18. Ronkainen J, Aro P, Storskrubb T, et al. Prevalence of Barrett's esophagus in the general population: an endoscopic study. Gastroenterology 2005;129:1825–31.

19. Rex DK, Cummings OW, Shaw M, et al. Screening for Barrett's esophagus in colonoscopy patients with and without heartburn. Gastroenterology 2003;125:1670–7.

20. Shaheen NJ, Crosby MA, Bozymski EM, et al. Is there publication bias in the reporting of cancer risk in Barrett's esophagus? Gastroenterology 2000;119:333–8.

21. Drewitz DJ, Sampliner RE, Garewal HS. The incidence of adenocarcinoma in Barrett's esophagus: a prospective study of 170 patients followed 4.8 years. Am J Gastroenterol 1997;92:212–5.

22. Provenzale D, Schmitt C, Wong JB. Barrett's esophagus: a new look at surveillance based on emerging estimates of cancer risk. Am J Gastroenterol 1999;94:2043–53.

23. Iftikhar SY, James PD, Steele RJ, et al. Length of Barrett's oesophagus: an important factor in the development of dysplasia and adenocarcinoma. Gut 1992;33:1155–8.

24. Weston AP, Krmpotich PT, Cherian R, et al. Prospective long-term endoscopic and histological follow-up of short segment Barrett's esophagus: comparison with traditional long segment Barrett's esophagus. Am J Gastroenterol 1997;92: 407–13.
25. Avidan B, Sonnenberg A, Schnell TG, et al. Hiatal hernia size, Barrett's length, and severity of acid reflux are all risk factors for esophageal adenocarcinoma. Am J Gastroenterol 2002;97:1930–6.
26. Rudolph RE, Vaughan TL, Storer BE, et al. Effect of segment length on risk for neoplastic progression in patients with Barrett esophagus. Ann Intern Med 2000;132:612–20.
27. Wani SB, Falk GW, Hall M, et al. Low risk of developing dysplasia and esophageal adenocarcinoma (EAC) in patients with non-dysplastic Barrett's esophagus (BE): results from a large, multicenter, cohort study. Gastroenterology 2010;138:475c.
28. Pohl H, Welch HG. The role of overdiagnosis and reclassification in the marked increase of esophageal adenocarcinoma incidence. J Natl Cancer Inst 2005; 97:142–6.
29. Shaheen NJ, Sharma P, Overholt BF, et al. Radiofrequency ablation in Barrett's esophagus with dysplasia. N Engl J Med 2009;360:2277–88.
30. Fleischer DE, Overholt BF, Sharma VK, et al. Endoscopic ablation of Barrett's esophagus: a multicenter study with 2.5-year follow-up. Gastrointest Endosc 2008;68:867–76.
31. Fleischer DE, Odze R, Overholt BF, et al. The case for endoscopic treatment of non-dysplastic and low-grade dysplastic Barrett's esophagus. Dig Dis Sci 2010;55:1918–31.

Barrett's Esophagus Surveillance: When, How Often, Does It Work?

Bryson W. Katona, MD, PhD[a], Gary W. Falk, MD, MS[b],*

KEYWORDS

- Barrett's esophagus • Endoscopic surveillance • Dysplasia
- Esophageal adenocarcinoma

THE CLINICAL PROBLEM OF ESOPHAGEAL ADENOCARCINOMA

Barrett's esophagus is a recognized risk factor for the development of esophageal adenocarcinoma. The incidence of this cancer has increased approximately 6-fold between 1975 and 2001, a rate greater than that of any other cancer in the United States during that time.[1] This increase has been accompanied by an increase in mortality rates from 2 to 15 deaths per million during that same time period.[1] Despite these alarming findings, the overall burden of esophageal adenocarcinoma remains low. It is estimated that there will be 16,640 new cases of esophageal cancer in the United States (of which more than half will be adenocarcinoma) accompanied by approximately 14,500 deaths in 2010.[2] Survival in esophageal adenocarcinoma is inversely related to the depth of invasion as well as lymph node metastases.[3,4] Patients with T1-stage disease have a survival rate of greater than 90% at 5 years, but this group represents less than 10% of patients undergoing esophagectomy in the United States.[3] Therefore, detection of adenocarcinoma at earlier stages has the potential to dramatically improve survival in these patients.[4]

The association of Barrett's esophagus with the development of adenocarcinoma, the often years-long stepwise progression of columnar metaplasia to adenocarcinoma, and the poor prognosis of advanced adenocarcinoma all make endoscopic surveillance an attractive option for Barrett's esophagus patients.[5] As such, regular endoscopic surveillance is recommended by all of the major American professional

---

Disclosures: Dr Gary Falk is a consultant for Genomic Health.
[a] Department of Internal Medicine, Hospital of the University of Pennsylvania, 3400 Spruce Street, 100 Centrex, Philadelphia, PA 19104, USA
[b] Division of Gastroenterology, Department of Internal Medicine, Hospital of the University of Pennsylvania, 3400 Spruce Street, 3rd Floor Ravdin Building, Philadelphia, PA 19104, USA
* Corresponding author.
E-mail address: gary.falk@uphs.upenn.edu

societies as well as other international gastroenterology organizations in an attempt to detect cancer at an early and potentially curable stage.[6–10]

WHO SHOULD UNDERGO SURVEILLANCE?

Only patients with a clear diagnosis of Barrett's esophagus are candidates for surveillance. The diagnosis of Barrett's esophagus is established if the squamocolumnar junction is displaced proximal to the gastroesophageal junction and intestinal metaplasia is detected by biopsy, although the need for intestinal metaplasia for the diagnosis has recently been questioned.[11] Recent evidence suggests that nongoblet columnar metaplasia demonstrates DNA content abnormalities indicative of neoplastic risk similar to those encountered in intestinal metaplasia, and the risk of developing esophageal adenocarcinoma is similar among patients with and without intestinal metaplasia.[12,13] The professional societies of North America all require intestinal metaplasia for the diagnosis of Barret esophagus whereas the British Society of Gastroenterology and a global consensus group do not require the presence of intestinal metaplasia for the diagnosis.[7,8,10,14,15] Currently, the issue of intestinal metaplasia versus columnar metaplasia as a diagnostic criterion for Barrett's esophagus remains unsettled.

Before entering into a surveillance program, patients should be advised about risks and benefits, including the limitations of surveillance endoscopy as well as the importance of adhering to appropriate surveillance intervals.[6] Other considerations include age less than 80 years, likelihood of survival over the next 5 years, and ability to tolerate either endoscopic or surgical interventions for early esophageal adenocarcinoma. Patients without documented Barrett's esophagus or in poor overall health will likely not benefit from endoscopic surveillance programs. Recent advances in endoscopic therapy with techniques, such as radiofrequency ablation and endoscopic mucosal resection, have the potential to change the inclusion criteria for Barrett's esophagus surveillance in the future. This may ultimately lead to application of surveillance programs to a wider population.

The number of individuals with Barrett's esophagus is sizable. It is estimated that Barrett's esophagus is found in approximately 5% to 15% of patients undergoing endoscopy for symptoms of gastroesophageal reflux disease.[16] Population-based studies suggest that the prevalence of Barrett's esophagus is approximately 1.3% to 1.6%.[17,18] A recent simulation model using the Surveillance, Epidemiology and End Result cancer registry estimated that the prevalence of Barrett's esophagus was 5.6% in the general population of the United States.[19] Using these data, the number of eligible patients for surveillance in the United States could range from 4 to 20 million individuals. The economic consequences of surveillance for this large a population are considerable, emphasizing the importance of developing more effective and selective surveillance programs than are currently in use.

HOW SHOULD SURVEILLANCE BE DONE?

The aim of surveillance is the detection of dysplasia or early cancer. Active inflammation makes it more difficult to distinguish dysplasia from reparative changes. As such, it is essential that surveillance endoscopy is only performed after any active inflammation related to gastroesophageal reflux disease is controlled with antisecretory therapy. The presence of ongoing erosive esophagitis is a contraindication to performing surveillance biopsies.

At the time of endoscopy, the esophagus should first be carefully examined with high-resolution white light endoscopy, with definition of appropriate landmarks, including the diaphragmatic hiatus, esophagogastric junction, and squamocolumnar junction before commencing biopsies.[20] It is still unclear how much enhanced imaging techniques add to careful inspection with high-resolution or high-definition white light endoscopy. Because the distribution of dysplastic mucosa and cancer is patchy in Barrett's esophagus, current guidelines suggest obtaining systematic four-quadrant biopsies at 2-cm intervals along the entire length of the Barrett segment commencing at the proximal margin of the gastric folds and continuing to the transition zone at the squamo-columnar junction.[7,21] The rationale for such a comprehensive biopsy program comes from the focal nature of dysplasia and the observation that high-grade dysplasia and early carcinoma in Barrett's esophagus often occur in the absence of endoscopic abnormalities.[21]

A systematic biopsy protocol detects more dysplasia and early cancer compared with ad hoc random biopsies.[22,23] Furthermore, the safety of systematic endoscopic biopsy protocols has been well demonstrated.[24] Subtle mucosal abnormalities, no matter how trivial, such as ulceration, erosion, plaque, nodule, stricture, or other luminal irregularity in the Barrett segment, should also be extensively biopsied, because there is an association of such lesions with underlying cancer.[25] Current guidelines recommend that mucosal abnormalities, especially in the setting of high-grade dysplasia, should undergo endoscopic mucosal resection.[7] Endoscopic mucosal resection changes the diagnosis in approximately 50% of patients compared with endoscopic biopsies, given the larger tissue sample available for review by a pathologist.[26] Interobserver agreement among pathologists is improved as well.[27]

There has been considerable debate over the years regarding the need for large particle (jumbo) forceps to obtain biopsies, a technique that requires passage of a therapeutic larger-caliber endoscope. Current guidelines suggest, however, that best available evidence does not support the routine use of the jumbo biopsy forceps. New large-capacity forceps that can be passed through the biopsy channel of standard-diameter endoscopes provides larger samples than standard large-capacity forceps and may increase the yield of dysplasia, thus providing a reasonable alternative approach.[28] The increasing importance of appropriately applied endoscopic mucosal resection, however, has changed biopsy sampling considerably and makes much of this debate of historical interest only.

There is some evidence that a smaller biopsy interval of 1 cm in addition to biopsies of visible lesions is more effective at detection of adenocarcinoma in patients with high-grade dysplasia, a method known as the Seattle protocol.[25] Although this protocol was considered ideal for patients with high-grade dysplasia, a recent comparison of the Seattle protocol with standard four-quadrant biopsies every 2 cm in a group of patients with high-grade dysplasia found that the detection of unsuspected cancer at the time of esophagectomy was no different between the two groups.[29] This intensive biopsy protocol has yet to be adopted into official surveillance guidelines. Furthermore, the widespread use of endoscopic mucosal resection in patients with high-grade dysplasia or early adenocarcinoma has changed the paradigm for these patients considerably.

Another available surveillance method is brush cytology.[30] Brush cytology is simpler and less expensive than endoscopic biopsy protocols and has the ability to sample more of the mucosal surface. One study found a 72% concordance rate between brush cytology specimens and simultaneous biopsies with cytology often demonstrating higher grades of dysplasia.[31] More recent work from the Cleveland Clinic demonstrated 95% specificity for brush cytology with 82% sensitivity for the detection of high-grade dysplasia or adenocarcinoma, but the sensitivity for low-grade dysplasia was only 31%.[32] Currently, cytology is not recommended as an appropriate surveillance technique. Cytology does have considerable potential as a platform for molecular biomarker techniques, however, such as fluorescence in situ hybridization, should they become validated.[33,34]

Once biopsy specimens are obtained, the samples are classified with a standard five-tier system as (1) negative for dysplasia, (2) indefinite for dysplasia, (3) low-grade dysplasia, (4) high-grade dysplasia, or (5) carcinoma. Any diagnosis of dysplasia should be confirmed by an expert gastrointestinal pathologist.[6–10] One report found that when low-grade dysplasia was a consensus diagnosis between two expert pathologists, there was a subsequent increased risk of further neoplastic transformation.[35] Furthermore, confirmation by expert pathologists often leads to downgrading of biopsies graded as low-grade dysplasia or high-grade dysplasia by general pathologists.[36] In one study, 64 of 71 (90%) samples of low-grade dysplasia were downgraded as were 11 of 23 (48%) samples of high-grade dysplasia.[36] Reasons for downgrading biopsies include ulceration, ongoing inflammation, and tangential sectioning of specimens.

HOW OFTEN SHOULD SURVEILLANCE BE PERFORMED?

Surveillance intervals, determined by the presence and grade of dysplasia, are based on the limited understanding of the biology of esophageal adenocarcinoma. These intervals, however, are arbitrary, have never been subject to a clinical trial, and likely never will be. Guidelines from the various professional societies are not in agreement on surveillance intervals. Surveillance every 3 years is recommended as adequate in patients without dysplasia after two negative examinations by both the American College of Gastroenterology and the American Society for Gastrointestinal Endoscopy (**Table 1**).[7,8] The American Gastroenterological Association recommends extending the surveillance interval up to 5 years whereas the British Society of Gastroenterology recommends continued surveillance at 2-year intervals in this setting.[6,10] Alternatively, the French Society of Digestive Endoscopy recommends intervals in patients without dysplasia based on the Barrett segment length (see **Table 1**).[9] A recent meta-analysis, however, showed that the risk of cancer was no different between short- and long-segment Barrett's esophagus.[37]

Table 1
Professional society guidelines for surveillance intervals in Barrett's esophagus patients with no dysplasia

Organization	Surveillance Interval
American College of Gastroenterology	Two EGDs in first year If negative for dysplasia, then every 3 years
American Gastroenterological Association	Two EGDs in first year If negative for dysplasia, then every 5 years
American Society for Gastrointestinal Endoscopy	Two EGDs in first year If negative for dysplasia, then every 3 years
British Society of Gastroenterology	Every 2 years
French Society of Digestive Endoscopy	Short-segment Barrett's esophagus (<3 cm)—every 5 years Long-segment Barrett's esophagus (3–6 cm)—every 3 years Long-segment Barrett's esophagus (>6 cm)—every 2 years

Abbreviation: EGD, esophagogastroduodenoscopy.
Data from Refs.[6–10]

If low-grade dysplasia is found, the diagnosis should first be confirmed by an expert gastrointestinal pathologist due to the marked interobserver variability in interpretation of these biopsies. These patients should also receive aggressive antisecretory therapy for reflux disease with a proton pump inhibitor to decrease the changes of regeneration that make pathologic interpretation of this category so difficult. Patients with confirmed low-grade dysplasia warrant shorter surveillance intervals and, therefore, more intensive monitoring. There is minor discord between the American organizations, with all three requiring at least one repeat endoscopy within 6 to 12 months after the initial diagnostic endoscopy (**Table 2**). Subsequent recommendations for follow-up intervals also vary between the American organizations (outlined in **Table 2**).[6–8] Both the British and French guidelines recommend a trial of aggressive acid suppression therapy for 1 to 2 months followed by repeat endoscopy (see **Table 2**).[9,10] If low-grade dysplasia persists after intensive acid suppression therapy, then the European guidelines suggest that follow-up endoscopies be performed every 6 months until two consecutive endoscopies demonstrate no dysplasia.[9,10] There is no agreement on the biopsy protocol to use, although a protocol of four-quadrant biopsies at 1-cm intervals as used for high-grade dysplasia makes sense to the authors. Endoscopic mucosal resection should be performed if any mucosal abnormality is present in these patients.

If high-grade dysplasia is found, the diagnosis should be confirmed by an experienced gastrointestinal pathologist. High-grade dysplasia is considered a threshold for intervention by both the American College of Gastroenterology and the French Society of Digestive Endoscopy after confirmation by repeat endoscopy within 2 to 3 months (**Table 3**).[7,9] A strategy of continued endoscopic surveillance in these patients may well be eclipsed by endoscopic intervention, and current guidelines may be out of date given the rapid evolution of endoscopic approaches. If continued

Table 2
Professional society guidelines for surveillance intervals in Barrett's esophagus patients with low-grade dysplasia

Organization	Surveillance Interval
American College of Gastroenterology	Repeat EGD in 6 months Then yearly EGD until no dysplasia for 2 years
American Gastroenterological Association	Repeat EGD within 1 year If LGD confirmed by two expert pathologists, then yearly EGD Otherwise, if disagreement, then every 2 years
American Society for Gastrointestinal Endoscopy	Repeat EGD in 6 months Additional EGD in 6 months, then yearly
British Society of Gastroenterology	Acid suppression for 8–12 weeks, then repeat EGD If LGD persists, EGDs every 6 months After two EGDs with no dysplasia, increase to every 2–3 years
French Society of Digestive Endoscopy	Double-dose PPI for 2 months, then repeat EGD If LGD persists, EGD at 6 months, 1 year and then yearly

Abbreviations: EGD, esophagogastroduodenoscopy; LGD, low-grade dysplasia; PPI, proton pump inhibitor.
Data from Refs. [6–10]

Table 3
Professional society guidelines for surveillance intervals in Barrett's esophagus patients with high-grade dysplasia

Organization	Surveillance Interval
American College of Gastroenterology	Repeat EGD in 3 months If HGD present, needs additional intervention
American Gastroenterological Association	Repeat EGD every 3 months 8 biopsies every 2 cm
American Society for Gastrointestinal Endoscopy	Repeat EGD every 3 months After 1 year, if two EGDs with no dysplasia, can lengthen interval
British Society of Gastroenterology	EGDs every 6 months if no additional interventions
French Society of Digestive Endoscopy	Double-dose PPI for 1–2 months, then repeat EGD If HGD persists, needs additional intervention

Abbreviations: EGD, esophagogastroduodenoscopy; HGD, high-grade dysplasia; PPI, proton pump inhibitor.
Data from Refs. [6–10]

surveillance is chosen, one proposed option is surveillance at 3-month intervals for 1 year.[38] If there is no high-grade dysplasia on two consecutive endoscopies for the first year, endoscopy frequency is lengthened to every 6 months for the second year then to annually thereafter as long as high-grade dysplasia is not encountered again. If high-grade dysplasia persists, then continued short-interval endoscopy is warranted.

Extent of high-grade dysplasia is thought by some investigators to be a risk factor for the subsequent development of adenocarcinoma.[39] There are currently no uniform criteria for defining the extent of high-grade dysplasia and there are conflicting data on the clinical significance of extent of high-grade dysplasia in biopsy specimens and risk for unsuspected carcinoma.[39,40] Mucosal abnormalities in patients with multifocal high-grade dysplasia may also be a risk factor for adenocarcinoma.[41,42]

DOES SURVEILLANCE ENDOSCOPY WORK?

Several observational studies suggest that patients with Barrett's esophagus in whom adenocarcinoma was detected in a surveillance program have their cancers detected at an earlier stage (**Fig. 1**), with markedly improved 5-year survival compared with similar patients not undergoing routine endoscopic surveillance (**Fig. 2**).[22,43–48] Furthermore, nodal involvement is far less likely in surveyed patients compared with nonsurveyed patients.[45] Because esophageal cancer survival is stage dependent, these studies suggest that survival may be enhanced by endoscopic surveillance. Several decision-analysis models support the concept of endoscopic surveillance.[49–51] The model of Provenzale and colleagues[49,51] suggests that surveillance every 5 years is the most effective strategy to increase both length and quality of life, whereas the model of Inadomi and colleagues[51] suggests that surveillance should be limited only to individuals with dysplasia at the time of initial endoscopy. Because most patients with Barrett's esophagus do not die from esophageal cancer, however, the entire concept of surveillance remains of uncertain benefit.[52] Design flaws, such as selection bias, healthy volunteer bias, lead time bias, and length time bias, are inherent in the observational studies that support endoscopic surveillance. Despite the

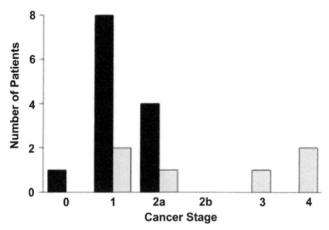

Fig. 1. Esophageal adenocarcinoma stage distribution. Stages of surveillance-detected cancers (*black bars*) versus nonsurveillance-detected cancers (*gray bars*). (*From* Corley DA, Levin TR, Habel LA, et al. Surveillance and survival in Barrett's adenocarcinomas: a population-based study. Gastroenterology 2002;122(3):633–40.)

concern regarding the esophageal cancer "epidemic," the overall burden of disease is limited in the Western world in comparison with other malignancies, such as colon cancer.

The ideal study to accurately determine if surveillance is an effective strategy in Barrett's esophagus would be a randomized controlled trial with a group of patients receiving surveillance and a second group not receiving any surveillance. The Barrett's Esophagus Surveillance Study (BOSS) trial in the United Kingdom is currently addressing this unmet need.[53] This study randomizes patients to receive either routine surveillance upper endoscopy every 2 years or upper endoscopy only as indicated by development of symptoms, with follow-up planned for 10 years.[53] Once completed, this trial will serve as an important benchmark for determining the benefit or lack thereof for Barrett's esophagus surveillance.

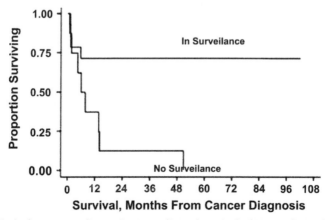

Fig. 2. Survival after cancer diagnosis. Age-adjusted survival after esophageal adenocarcinoma diagnosis in patients receiving surveillance versus no surveillance. (*From* Corley DA, Levin TR, Habel LA, et al. Surveillance and survival in Barrett's adenocarcinomas: a population-based study. Gastroenterology 2002;122(3):633–40.)

ARE SURVEILLANCE GUIDELINES FOLLOWED BY GASTROENTEROLOGISTS?

Surveillance is favored by the majority of gastroenterologists, with 94% of those surveyed by the British Society of Gastroenterology offering surveillance for Barrett's esophagus patients.[54] Other survey studies report that approximately 84% to 96% of physicians perform surveillance in Barrett's esophagus patients.[55,56] Despite the existence of professional society guidelines for surveillance as well as statistics on this topic (discussed previously), these guidelines are not always followed in clinical practice.

Several studies have found that surveillance intervals in clinical practice are highly variable and often shorter than recommended.[54,57,58] One recent study demonstrated that nearly 50% of physicians performed surveillance every 1 to 2 years in patients with no dysplasia whereas more than 60% performed surveillance every 6 months or less for patients with documented low-grade dysplasia.[57] Other work has demonstrated more variation in low-grade dysplasia surveillance intervals when compared with patients with no dysplasia or high-grade dysplasia.[59] This observation, however, may also be a reflection of confusion based on the lack of agreement among the various practice guidelines (discussed previously).[6-10]

A variety of physician factors may also play a role in the variable adherence to practice guidelines. Gastroenterologists over age 45 and those receiving primarily fee-for-service both used shorter surveillance intervals than their younger, salaried counterparts.[60] One recent retrospective analysis, however, found that shorter interval surveillance for low-grade dysplasia was associated with increased detection of high-grade dysplasia and esophageal cancer.[58]

Use of four-quadrant biopsies every 2 cm is routinely recommended by practice guidelines, yet adherence to this recommendation is problematic. Surveys suggest that only 41% to 59% of gastroenterologists surveyed consistently used the four-quadrant biopsy method of surveillance.[54,57,61,62] Adherence to the four-quadrant biopsy method was more prevalent with shorter segments of Barrett's esophagus.[63,64] A more recent study also confirmed decreased biopsy adherence with increased Barrett segment length (**Fig. 3**) and demonstrated that nonadherence to the surveillance guidelines was associated with a decreased detection of dysplasia (**Fig. 4**).[62] Lastly, confirmation of dysplasia by two expert pathologists is also problematic. Only half of endoscopists surveyed used two expert pathologists to review cases of high-grade dysplasia.[54,57] Furthermore, a French study found an even lower use rate, with only 29% of gastroenterologists surveyed obtaining expert confirmation of dysplasia by two or more pathologists.[61]

HOW CAN ADHERENCE TO SURVEILLANCE GUIDELINES BE IMPROVED?

Although many studies have documented the problems with adherence to surveillance guidelines, 92% of gastroenterologists indicated that their poor adherence was due to lack of solid evidence supporting the effectiveness of surveillance, such as a randomized controlled trial.[57] A variety of options have been explored to improve adherence to surveillance guidelines, including the institution of a structured protocol for surveillance, providing guidelines to physicians, and the use of surveillance coordinators.[57,65-67]

A structured surveillance protocol was instituted at centers participating in the Aspirin Esomeprazole Chemoprevention Trial (AspECT).[57] Institution of this structured protocol led to significant improvement in adherence to guidelines for the management of low-grade dysplasia, increased surveillance of short-segment Barrett's esophagus, increased use of the four-quadrant biopsy technique, and increased number of biopsy specimens submitted for each patient (**Table 4**).[57] A more recent study, also looking at implementation of a structured surveillance program, found improvement in adherence

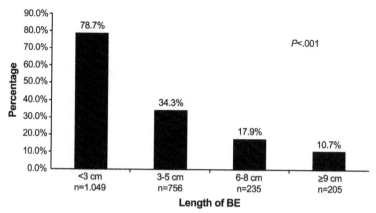

Fig. 3. Surveillance adherence by Barrett length. Adherence by gastroenterologists to the Seattle biopsy protocol by Barrett segment length. BE, Barrett's esophagus. (*From* Abrams JA, Kapel RC, Lindberg GM, et al. Adherence to biopsy guidelines for Barrett's esophagus surveillance in the community setting in the United States. Clin Gastroenterol Hepatol 2009;7:736–42.)

to endoscopic surveillance intervals, with 94% of patients receiving endoscopy at the appropriate interval.[65] In this study, four-quadrant biopsies every 2 cm were also performed during 90% of endoscopies,[65] which was a marked improvement over previous data.[54,57,61] Although a structured surveillance protocol improves adherence to surveillance recommendations, implementation requires additional administrative support as

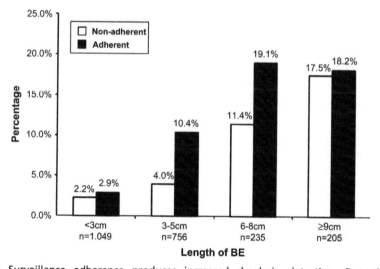

Fig. 4. Surveillance adherence produces increased dysplasia detection. Detection of dysplasia (low-grade dysplasia, high-grade dysplasia, or esophageal adenocarcinoma) in cases adherent and nonadherent to the Seattle biopsy protocol. Mantel-Haenszel test summary odds ratio of 0.53 (95% CI, 0.35–0.82). BE, Barrett's esophagus. (*From* Abrams JA, Kapel RC, Lindberg GM, et al. Adherence to biopsy guidelines for Barrett's esophagus surveillance in the community setting in the United States. Clin Gastroenterol Hepatol 2009;7:736–42.)

well as increased pathologic and endoscopic resources.[65] It remains to be seen if improved adherence to surveillance guidelines will ultimately improve important clinical outcomes, such as survival, in these patients.

Another potential approach to improving physician adherence is dissemination of both surveillance guidelines and/or statistical data from an audit of physician adherence to current guidelines. Both of these interventions did not seem to change clinical practice.[66] When disseminated guidelines were combined, however, in a multifaceted intervention with conferences and surveillance reminders, compliance with both appropriate biopsy technique and surveillance intervals were significantly increased.[67] Finally, introduction of surveillance coordinators who oversee a center's surveillance program may also improve adherence to guidelines.[66] Specifically, a recent prospective audit showed that coordinators increased adherence to surveillance intervals from 17% to 92% and similarly increased the number of endoscopies, where sufficient biopsies were obtained from 45% to 83%.[66]

WHAT IS THE ECONOMIC BURDEN OF BARRETT'S ESOPHAGUS SURVEILLANCE PROGRAMS AND IS IT WORTH IT?

Barrett surveillance programs are endoscopically intensive requiring significant resources, and the vast majority of patients with Barrett's esophagus patients die of causes other than adenocarcinoma.[68] Therefore, it is appropriate to analyze whether or not these programs are cost effective. A recent study in the United Kingdom compared a Barrett's esophagus surveillance program consisting of patients who had annual endoscopy with control patients who presented with esophageal adenocarcinoma.[69] The additional cost of Barrett surveillance was £4493 (approximately $6700) per life year gained.[69] A separate study found a cost of $10,440 per quality-adjusted life year in Barrett's esophagus patients with known dysplasia who were in

Table 4
Improved surveillance adherence in the AspECT Trial. Summary of Barrett's surveillance adherence before and after initiation of AspECT study

	Before AspECT Initiation	After AspECT Initiation	Change and Significance
Adherence to guidelines for management of LGD	48%	63%	↑P<0.01
Referral of HGD for surgical resection	75%	60%	↓P < 0.01
Identification of HH by objective criteria	54	70	↑P < 0.01
Surveillance of all short-segment BE cases (<2-cm length)	6%	60%	↑P < 0.01
Use of 4-quadrant biopsy protocol	32%	86%	↑P < 0.01
No. of biopsies/cm BE	1.54 (SD 0.64)	2.12 (SD 1.04)	↑P < 0.002

Abbreviations: LGD, low grade dysplasia; HGD, high grade dysplasia; HH, hiatal hernia; BE, Barrett's esophagus.
From Das D, Ishaq S, Harrison R, et al. Management of Barrett's esophagus in the UK: overtreated and underbiopsied but improved by the introduction of a national randomized trial. Am J Gastroenterol 2008;103(5):1079–89; with permission.

a surveillance program.[51] This is a reasonable figure when compared with other commonly used thresholds for cost-effectiveness that range between $20,000 and $85,000 per quality-adjusted life year.[70] This figure increases significantly, however, for Barrett's esophagus patients with no known dysplasia, leading the authors to question the expense of surveillance in this group, even at 5-year intervals.[51] Furthermore, a recent meta-analysis questioned the cost-effectiveness of Barrett's esophagus surveillance because of the low risk of malignant progression[68] in conjunction with the lack of change in life expectancy in Barrett's esophagus patients when compared with control populations.[71] Other work has examined the cost-effectiveness of different intervals of surveillance, with surveillance at 5-year intervals more cost effective than surveillance at 1- to 4-year intervals.[49] In the end, the majority of studies suggest that Barrett's esophagus surveillance is a cost-effective strategy.[50] Better risk stratification tools are urgently needed, however, to improve flaws inherent in the current approach to surveillance.[68]

HOW CAN SURVEILLANCE BE IMPROVED?

Currently, all Barrett's esophagus patients are handled in a similar fashion unless dysplasia is present. Because most patients do not have dysplasia and never develop cancer, it is necessary to make surveillance techniques more effective by either sampling larger areas of Barrett mucosa, targeting biopsies to areas with a higher probability of harboring dysplasia, or developing risk stratification tools to allow concentrating efforts on individuals at greatest risk while decreasing the frequency and intensity of surveillance in individuals at lower risk. New imaging techniques, such as high-definition white light, magnification, narrow band imaging, autofluorescence imaging, and confocal microscopy, are currently being investigated to aid in better detection of dysplasia or adenocarcinoma.[72] Improved methods for tissue sampling are still needed, although endoscopic mucosal resection has already made a difference in this regard. Further discussion of these specific techniques is beyond the scope of this article.

Surveillance could also be improved through the development of a better system for risk stratification of Barrett's esophagus patients, using both clinical and biologic markers. Clinical risk factors for development of high-grade dysplasia or adenocarcinoma include male gender, older age, white race, hiatal hernia size, length of the Barrett segment, smoking, and body mass index, with a focus on male pattern central obesity.[73] There are also some known protective factors, including Helicobacter pylori infection, aspirin/nonsteroidal anti-inflammatory drugs, and increased fruit and vegetable intake.[73] Currently, dysplasia remains the only factor in clinical practice that increases the risk of adenocarcinoma. Biomarkers that may define individuals at increased risk of cancer are still urgently needed. Although several studies have provided the conceptual framework for biomarkers of increased risk, none of biomarkers studied to date is ready for clinical practice. Detailed discussion of this topic is beyond the scope of this article. An improved system of risk stratification (using the criteria discussed previously) would ideally provide surveillance for the highest-risk Barrett's esophagus patients who would receive a true mortality benefit from a surveillance program. It is likely that in the future, the best predictor for the development of high-grade dysplasia or adenocarcinoma will be a combination of clinical, demographic, histologic, genetic, and epigenetic data. Any new risk stratification tool, however, would have to undergo thorough testing before implementation to determine if it is more effective than the current approach to Barrett's esophagus surveillance.

SUMMARY

Barrett's esophagus predisposes patients to the development of adenocarcinoma. Endoscopic surveillance of these patients is uniformly recommended, but the professional society guidelines are not in agreement and surveillance is not supported by definitive randomized controlled trials. Nonetheless, current observational studies suggest that surveillance of Barrett's esophagus is appropriate and cost effective and results in improved survival in surveillance-detected cancers compared with cancers not detected in surveillance. Surveillance techniques and intervals continue to evolve as better techniques for tissue visualization and sampling are developed and more effective risk stratification models are created. Long-term studies are still needed to determine which patients benefit most from ongoing surveillance.

REFERENCES

1. Pohl H, Welch HG. The role of overdiagnosis and reclassification in the marked increase of esophageal adenocarcinoma incidence. J Natl Cancer Inst 2005;97(2):142–6.
2. Jemal A, Siegel R, Xu J, et al. Cancer Statistics, 2010. CA Cancer J Clin 2010;60: 277–300.
3. Visbal AL, Allen MS, Miller DL, et al. Ivor Lewis esophagogastrectomy for esophageal cancer. Ann Thorac Surg 2001;71(6):1803–8.
4. Menke-Pluymers MB, Schoute NW, Mulder AH, et al. Outcome of surgical treatment of adenocarcinoma in Barrett's oesophagus. Gut 1992;33(11):1454–8.
5. Tomizawa Y, Wang KK. Screening, surveillance, and prevention for esophageal cancer. Gastroenterol Clin North Am 2009;38(1):59–73, viii.
6. Wang KK, Wongkeesong M, Buttar NS. American Gastroenterological Association medical position statement: role of the gastroenterologist in the management of esophageal carcinoma. Gastroenterology 2005;128(5):1468–70.
7. Wang KK, Sampliner RE. Updated guidelines 2008 for the diagnosis, surveillance and therapy of Barrett's esophagus. Am J Gastroenterol 2008;103(3):788–97.
8. Hirota WK, Zuckerman MJ, Adler DG, et al. ASGE guideline: the role of endoscopy in the surveillance of premalignant conditions of the upper GI tract. Gastrointest Endosc 2006;63(4):570–80.
9. Boyer J, Laugier R, Chemali M, et al. French Society of Digestive Endoscopy SFED guideline: monitoring of patients with Barrett's esophagus. Endoscopy 2007;39(9):840–2.
10. British Society of Gastroenterology. Guidelines for the diagnosis and management of Barrett's columnar-lined oesophagus. Available at: http://www.bsg.org.uk. Accessed August 15, 2010.
11. Riddell RH, Odze RD. Definition of Barrett's esophagus: time for a rethink—is intestinal metaplasia dead? Am J Gastroenterol 2009;104(10):2588–94.
12. Kelty CJ, Gough MD, Van Wyk Q, et al. Barrett's oesophagus: intestinal metaplasia is not essential for cancer risk. Scand J Gastroenterol 2007;42(11):1271–4.
13. Liu W, Hahn H, Odze RD, et al. Metaplastic esophageal columnar epithelium without goblet cells shows DNA content abnormalities similar to goblet cell-containing epithelium. Am J Gastroenterol 2009;104(4):816–24.
14. Vakil N, van Zanten SV, Kahrilas P, et al. The Montreal definition and classification of gastroesophageal reflux disease: a global evidence-based consensus. Am J Gastroenterol 2006;101(8):1900–20 [quiz: 1943].
15. Wang KK, Wongkeesong M, Buttar NS. American Gastroenterological Association technical review on the role of the gastroenterologist in the management of esophageal carcinoma. Gastroenterology 2005;128(5):1471–505.

16. Westhoff B, Brotze S, Weston A, et al. The frequency of Barrett's esophagus in high-risk patients with chronic GERD. Gastrointest Endosc 2005;61(2):226–31.
17. Ronkainen J, Aro P, Storskrubb T, et al. Prevalence of Barrett's esophagus in the general population: an endoscopic study. Gastroenterology 2005;129(6):1825–31.
18. Zagari RM, Fuccio L, Wallander MA, et al. Gastro-oesophageal reflux symptoms, oesophagitis and Barrett's oesophagus in the general population: the Loiano-Monghidoro study. Gut 2008;57(10):1354–9.
19. Hayeck TJ, Kong CY, Spechler SJ, et al. The prevalence of Barrett's esophagus in the US: estimates from a simulation model confirmed by SEER data. Dis Esophagus 2010;23:451–7.
20. Falk GW. Screening and surveillance of barrett's esophagus. In: Sharma P, Sampliner RE, editors. Barrett's esophagus and esophageal adenocarcinoma. Malden (MA): Blackwell Science; 2001. p. 89–105.
21. Cameron AJ, Carpenter HA. Barrett's esophagus, high-grade dysplasia, and early adenocarcinoma: a pathological study. Am J Gastroenterol 1997;92(4):586–91.
22. Fitzgerald RC, Saeed IT, Khoo D, et al. Rigorous surveillance protocol increases detection of curable cancers associated with Barrett's esophagus. Dig Dis Sci 2001;46(9):1892–8.
23. Abela JE, Going JJ, Mackenzie JF, et al. Systematic four-quadrant biopsy detects Barrett's dysplasia in more patients than nonsystematic biopsy. Am J Gastroenterol 2008;103(4):850–5.
24. Levine DS, Blount PL, Rudolph RE, et al. Safety of a systematic endoscopic biopsy protocol in patients with Barrett's esophagus. Am J Gastroenterol 2000; 95(5):1152–7.
25. Reid BJ, Blount PL, Feng Z, et al. Optimizing endoscopic biopsy detection of early cancers in Barrett's high-grade dysplasia. Am J Gastroenterol 2000; 95(11):3089–96.
26. Peters FP, Brakenhoff KP, Curvers WL, et al. Histologic evaluation of resection specimens obtained at 293 endoscopic resections in Barrett's esophagus. Gastrointest Endosc 2008;67(4):604–9.
27. Mino-Kenudson M, Hull MJ, Brown I, et al. EMR for Barrett's esophagus-related superficial neoplasms offers better diagnostic reproducibility than mucosal biopsy. Gastrointest Endosc 2007;66(4):660–6.
28. Komanduri S, Swanson G, Keefer L, et al. Use of a new jumbo forceps improves tissue acquisition of Barrett's esophagus surveillance biopsies. Gastrointest Endosc 2009;70(6):1072–8, e1071.
29. Kariv R, Plesec TP, Goldblum JR, et al. The Seattle protocol does not more reliably predict the detection of cancer at the time of esophagectomy than a less intensive surveillance protocol. Clin Gastroenterol Hepatol 2009;7(6):653–8 [quiz: 606].
30. Robey SS, Hamilton SR, Gupta PK, et al. Diagnostic value of cytopathology in Barrett esophagus and associated carcinoma. Am J Clin Pathol 1988;89(4):493–8.
31. Geisinger KR, Teot LA, Richter JE. A comparative cytopathologic and histologic study of atypia, dysplasia, and adenocarcinoma in Barrett's esophagus. Cancer 1992;69(1):8–16.
32. Kumaravel A, Lopez R, Brainard J, et al. Brush cytology versus endoscopic biopsy for the surveillance of Barrett's esophagus. Endoscopy 2010;42:800–5.
33. Falk GW, Skacel M, Gramlich TL, et al. Fluorescence in situ hybridization of cytologic specimens from Barrett's esophagus: a pilot feasibility study. Gastrointest Endosc 2004;60(2):280–4.
34. Fritcher EG, Brankley SM, Kipp BR, et al. A comparison of conventional cytology, DNA ploidy analysis, and fluorescence in situ hybridization for the detection of

dysplasia and adenocarcinoma in patients with Barrett's esophagus. Hum Pathol 2008;39(8):1128–35.

35. Skacel M, Petras RE, Gramlich TL, et al. The diagnosis of low-grade dysplasia in Barrett's esophagus and its implications for disease progression. Am J Gastroenterol 2000;95(12):3383–7.

36. Baak JP, ten Kate FJ, Offerhaus GJ, et al. Routine morphometrical analysis can improve reproducibility of dysplasia grade in Barrett's oesophagus surveillance biopsies. J Clin Pathol 2002;55(12):910–6.

37. Thomas T, Abrams KR, De Caestecker JS, et al. Meta analysis: cancer risk in Barrett's oesophagus. Aliment Pharmacol Ther 2007;26(11–12):1465–77.

38. Schnell TG, Sontag SJ, Chejfec G, et al. Long-term nonsurgical management of Barrett's esophagus with high-grade dysplasia. Gastroenterology 2001;120(7): 1607–19.

39. Buttar NS, Wang KK, Sebo TJ, et al. Extent of high-grade dysplasia in Barrett's esophagus correlates with risk of adenocarcinoma. Gastroenterology 2001; 120(7):1630–9.

40. Dar MS, Goldblum JR, Rice TW, et al. Can extent of high grade dysplasia in Barrett's oesophagus predict the presence of adenocarcinoma at oesophagectomy? Gut 2003;52(4):486–9.

41. Tharavej C, Hagen JA, Peters JH, et al. Predictive factors of coexisting cancer in Barrett's high-grade dysplasia. Surg Endosc 2006;20(3):439–43.

42. Nigro JJ, Hagen JA, DeMeester TR, et al. Occult esophageal adenocarcinoma: extent of disease and implications for effective therapy. Ann Surg 1999;230(3): 433–8 [discussion: 438–40].

43. Incarbone R, Bonavina L, Saino G, et al. Outcome of esophageal adenocarcinoma detected during endoscopic biopsy surveillance for Barrett's esophagus. Surg Endosc 2002;16(2):263–6.

44. Ferguson MK, Durkin A. Long-term survival after esophagectomy for Barrett's adenocarcinoma in endoscopically surveyed and nonsurveyed patients. J Gastrointest Surg 2002;6(1):29–35 [discussion: 36].

45. van Sandick JW, van Lanschot JJ, Kuiken BW, et al. Impact of endoscopic biopsy surveillance of Barrett's oesophagus on pathological stage and clinical outcome of Barrett's carcinoma. Gut 1998;43(2):216–22.

46. Peters JH, Clark GW, Ireland AP, et al. Outcome of adenocarcinoma arising in Barrett's esophagus in endoscopically surveyed and nonsurveyed patients. J Thorac Cardiovasc Surg 1994;108(5):813–21 [discussion: 821–2].

47. Corley DA, Levin TR, Habel LA, et al. Surveillance and survival in Barrett's adenocarcinomas: a population-based study. Gastroenterology 2002;122(3):633–40.

48. Fountoulakis A, Zafirellis KD, Dolan K, et al. Effect of surveillance of Barrett's oesophagus on the clinical outcome of oesophageal cancer. Br J Surg 2004; 91(8):997–1003.

49. Provenzale D, Schmitt C, Wong JB. Barrett's esophagus: a new look at surveillance based on emerging estimates of cancer risk. Am J Gastroenterol 1999; 94(8):2043–53.

50. Sonnenberg A, Soni A, Sampliner RE. Medical decision analysis of endoscopic surveillance of Barrett's oesophagus to prevent oesophageal adenocarcinoma. Aliment Pharmacol Ther 2002;16(1):41–50.

51. Inadomi JM, Sampliner R, Lagergren J, et al. Screening and surveillance for Barrett esophagus in high-risk groups: a cost-utility analysis. Ann Intern Med 2003;138(3):176–86.

52. Conio M, Blanchi S, Lapertosa G, et al. Long-term endoscopic surveillance of patients with Barrett's esophagus. Incidence of dysplasia and adenocarcinoma: a prospective study. Am J Gastroenterol 2003;98(9):1931–9.
53. Jankowski J, Barr H. Improving surveillance for Barrett's oesophagus: AspECT and BOSS trials provide an evidence base. BMJ 2006;332(7556):1512.
54. Mandal A, Playford RJ, Wicks AC. Current practice in surveillance strategy for patients with Barrett's oesophagus in the UK. Aliment Pharmacol Ther 2003; 17(10):1319–24.
55. van Sandick JW, Bartelsman JF, van Lanschot JJ, et al. Surveillance of Barrett's oesophagus: physicians' practices and review of current guidelines. Eur J Gastroenterol Hepatol 2000;12(1):111–7.
56. Falk GW, Ours TM, Richter JE. Practice patterns for surveillance of Barrett's esophagus in the united states. Gastrointest Endosc 2000;52(2):197–203.
57. Das D, Ishaq S, Harrison R, et al. Management of Barrett's esophagus in the UK: overtreated and underbiopsied but improved by the introduction of a national randomized trial. Am J Gastroenterol 2008;103(5):1079–89.
58. Ramus JR, Gatenby PA, Caygill CP, et al. Surveillance of Barrett's columnar-lined oesophagus in the UK: endoscopic intervals and frequency of detection of dysplasia. Eur J Gastroenterol Hepatol 2009;21(6):636–41.
59. Ramus JR, Caygill CP, Gatenby PA, et al. Current united kingdom practice in the diagnosis and management of columnar-lined oesophagus: results of the united kingdom national barrett's oesophagus registry endoscopist questionnaire. Eur J Cancer Prev 2008;17(5):422–5.
60. Gross CP, Canto MI, Hixson J, et al. Management of Barrett's esophagus: a national study of practice patterns and their cost implications. Am J Gastroenterol 1999;94(12):3440–7.
61. Amamra N, Touzet S, Colin C, et al. Current practice compared with the international guidelines: endoscopic surveillance of Barrett's esophagus. J Eval Clin Pract 2007;13(5):789–94.
62. Abrams JA, Kapel RC, Lindberg GM, et al. Adherence to biopsy guidelines for Barrett's esophagus surveillance in the community setting in the United States. Clin Gastroenterol Hepatol 2009;7(7):736–42 [quiz: 710].
63. Ramnath G, Bampton P. Surveillance for Barrett's oesophagus: if you do it, do it properly. Med J Aust 2004;180(3):139–40.
64. Curvers WL, Peters FP, Elzer B, et al. Quality of Barrett's surveillance in The Netherlands: a standardized review of endoscopy and pathology reports. Eur J Gastroenterol Hepatol 2008;20(7):601–7.
65. Bright T, Schloithe A, Bull JA, et al. Outcome of endoscopy surveillance for Barrett's oesophagus. ANZ J Surg 2009;79(11):812–6.
66. Bampton PA, Schloithe A, Bull J, et al. Improving surveillance for Barrett's oesophagus. BMJ 2006;332(7553):1320–3.
67. Amamra N, Touzet S, Colin C, et al. Impact of guidelines for endoscopy in patients with Barrett's esophagus: a multifaceted interventional study. Gastroenterol Clin Biol 2009;33(6-7):470–7.
68. Sikkema M, de Jonge PJ, Steyerberg EW, et al. Risk of esophageal adenocarcinoma and mortality in patients with Barrett's esophagus: a systematic review and meta-analysis. Clin Gastroenterol Hepatol 2010;8(3):235–44 [quiz: e232].
69. Roberts KJ, Harper E, Alderson D, et al. Long-term survival and cost analysis of an annual Barrett's surveillance programme. Eur J Gastroenterol Hepatol 2010; 22(4):399–403.

70. Evans C, Tavakoli M, Crawford B. Use of quality adjusted life years and life years gained as benchmarks in economic evaluations: a critical appraisal. Health Care Manag Sci 2004;7(1):43–9.

71. Eckardt VF, Kanzler G, Bernhard G. Life expectancy and cancer risk in patients with Barrett's esophagus: a prospective controlled investigation. Am J Med 2001; 111(1):33–7.

72. Sharma P. Clinical practice. Barrett's esophagus. N Engl J Med 2009;361(26): 2548–56.

73. Falk GW. Risk factors for esophageal cancer development. Surg Oncol Clin N Am 2009;18(3):469–85.

Biology of Barrett's Esophagus and Esophageal Adenocarcinoma

David H. Wang, MD, PhD[a,b,c], Rhonda F. Souza, MD[a,b],*

KEYWORDS

- Barrett's esophagus • Metaplasia
- Esophageal adenocarcinoma

Although overall cancer incidence in the United States has decreased in recent years,[1] the number of new cases of esophageal cancer is increasing.[2] According to American Cancer Society estimates, there were 16,470 new cases and 14,530 deaths in this country in 2009 from esophageal cancer.[3] Esophageal cancer has 2 main histologic subtypes: squamous cell carcinoma and adenocarcinoma. In the west, the incidence of the squamous cell carcinoma has remained stable or decreased since the 1970s; the incidence of adenocarcinoma has risen steadily during the same time period.[2] Esophageal adenocarcinoma has now become the more prevalent histologic subtype in the United States.[2]

Esophageal adenocarcinoma typically arises in the distal one-third of the esophagus, and its main risk factors are gastroesophageal reflux disease (GERD) and Barrett's esophagus. For patients with Barrett's esophagus, endoscopic surveillance to detect dysplasia is the primary strategy recommended to decrease morbidity and mortality from esophageal adenocarcinoma.[4] This strategy has not proved effective, as shown by the increasing incidence of esophageal adenocarcinoma and the results of a recent study showing that most patients with this cancer have no prior diagnosis of Barrett's esophagus and, therefore, are not enrolled in surveillance programs.[5]

This work was supported by the Office of Medical Research, Department of Veterans Affairs (R.F.S., D.H.W.) and the National Institutes of Health (F32-CA123945 to D.H.W. and R01-DK63621 & R01-CA134571 to R.F.S.).
The authors have nothing to disclose.
[a] Department of Medicine, Veterans Affairs North Texas Health Care System and the University of Texas Southwestern Medical School, 5323 Harry Hines Boulevard, Dallas, TX 75390, USA
[b] Harold C. Simmons Comprehensive Cancer Center, University of Texas Southwestern Medical Center at Dallas, 5323 Harry Hines Boulevard, Dallas, TX 75390, USA
[c] Division of Hematology-Oncology (111C), Dallas VA Medical Center, 4500 South Lancaster Road, Dallas, TX 75216, USA
* Corresponding author. Division of Gastroenterology (111B1), Dallas VA Medical Center, 4500 South Lancaster Road, Dallas, TX 75216.
E-mail address: rhonda.souza@utsouthwestern.edu

Basic investigations that have defined the genetic events underlying colonic carcinogenesis have led to effective strategies for the management and prevention of colorectal cancer.[6] Analogously, it is important to understand the molecular carcinogenesis of Barrett's esophagus to identify specific targets to guide the development of effective diagnostic strategies and novel therapeutic agents. To do this, the molecular events that lead to the replacement of normal esophageal squamous cells by metaplastic Barrett cells must first be understood. Building on this understanding, we can appreciate how the genetic abnormalities acquired by metaplastic Barrett cells disrupt their normal properties so they can take on the morphologic and physiologic features of dysplasia and cancer. This report provides a conceptual basis for how normal esophageal squamous cells undergo columnar metaplasia and how metaplastic Barrett cells progress to dysplasia and carcinoma. Some of the main genetic alterations involved in the development and neoplastic progression of Barrett's esophagus are reviewed; however, these represent a fraction of the genetic changes required for the making of Barrett metaplasia, dysplasia, and esophageal adenocarcinoma.

THE MAKING OF BARRETT METAPLASIA

Most, if not all, esophageal adenocarcinomas arise from Barrett's esophagus, the condition in which the normal squamous cells lining the distal esophagus are replaced by intestinal-type columnar cells.[7] Barrett's esophagus develops through the process of metaplasia, the replacement of one adult cell type by another. Metaplasia is believed to arise as a protective response to chronic tissue inflammation,[8] which in the esophagus is believed to be caused by GERD. Barrett metaplasia can result from either fully differentiated esophageal squamous cells changing directly into intestinal-type columnar cells or from changing the differentiation pattern of esophageal stem cells.[8]

METAPLASIA THROUGH TRANSDIFFERENTIATION

Transdifferentiation is the switch of one fully differentiated cell type directly into another. In general, this switch occurs between cell phenotypes that were present in the organ during embryonic development.[8] During embryogenesis, the esophagus is initially lined by ciliated columnar cells, which are replaced by stratified squamous cells as maturation proceeds (**Fig. 1**).[9,10] Data from ex vivo organ cultures of embryonic mouse esophagus demonstrate direct conversion of the columnar cells lining the esophagus into squamous cells, a process found to be independent of cell proliferation or apoptosis.[11] In theory, a reversal of this normal developmental switch in cell phenotype may occur during the formation of Barrett metaplasia. In support of this hypothesis, studies using scanning electron microscopy have demonstrated a distinctive cell at the squamocolumnar junction in Barrett mucosa that expresses cytokeratin markers and demonstrates morphologic features of both squamous and columnar epithelium; moreover, this distinctive cell has not been detected at the squamocolumnar junction in patients without Barrett mucosa.[12] Once Barrett metaplasia is established, the epithelium must undergo maintenance and self-renewal, processes that are not explained by the transdifferentiation hypothesis, however.

METAPLASIA THROUGH STEM CELLS

Stem cells can proliferate, self-renew, give rise to a variety of cell types, and regenerate tissue after injury.[13] A stem cell origin would account for the persistence and maintenance of Barrett epithelium and could explain the predisposition of this tissue

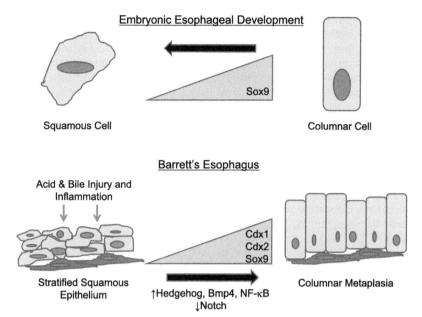

Fig. 1. Phenotypic changes in esophageal epithelium occur during normal development and Barrett's esophagus. During esophageal development (*top*), the embryonic esophagus is initially lined by columnar epithelial cells expressing the transcription factor Sox9. As the embryo matures, the esophageal epithelium transitions into a stratified squamous epithelium that does not express Sox9. In Barrett's esophagus (*bottom*), the stratified squamous epithelium is exposed to acid and bile acids. The ensuing inflammation and injury repair response activate signaling pathways such as Hedgehog, Bmp4, and NF-κB and downregulate Notch signaling. These signals lead to increased expression of Cdx1, Cdx2, and Sox9, which induces columnar metaplasia.

to neoplastic transformation. The stem cell for Barrett's esophagus may reside in the esophagus itself or originate in the bone marrow. During development, tracheo-esophageal progenitor cells express p63, a homolog of p53.[14] As the esophageal lining forms, p63+ progenitor cells differentiate into ciliated columnar cells that lack p63 expression.[14] After stratified squamous epithelium replaces the ciliated columnar epithelium, cells in the proliferative basal layer of the squamous epithelium continue to stain strongly for p63, whereas cells in the fully differentiated more superficial layers demonstrate no p63 staining.[14] In mice null for p63, the esophagi completely lack stratified epithelium and are lined by simple columnar epithelium, suggesting that p63+ cells are necessary to establish a stratified squamous epithelium.[14] Barrett epithelium has been found to lack immunostaining for p63, suggesting that the Barrett stem cell differs from the p63+ embryonic esophageal progenitor cell and the adult, squamous esophageal stem cell.[14,15] These findings do not eliminate the possibility that the stem cells for Barrett metaplasia reside in esophageal submucosal glands or in glands of the gastric cardia, adjacent to the gastroesophageal junction, as has been suggested by some investigators.[16,17]

A second potential source of stem cells for the esophagus is the bone marrow. In mice treated with high-dose irradiation to induce esophagitis, injection of either esophageal progenitor cells or bone marrow cells was able to repair the injured esophagus through regeneration of new squamous cells.[18] Using a rat model of severe reflux esophagitis, our group investigated the possibility that bone marrow cells can give rise to metaplastic Barrett epithelium. Female rats were lethally irradiated and then rescued with bone marrow from male donor rats. An esophagojejunostomy was then performed on the female rats to induce the reflux of both acid and bile salts.[19] Eight weeks after surgery, the esophagi of the female rats contained squamous and metaplastic cells with a Y chromosome, suggesting that bone marrow cells can hone to the esophagus and give rise to both squamous and columnar epithelium. In humans, cells from male donors have been found within the gastrointestinal tract of female patients who have undergone bone marrow transplant.[20]

Regardless of where the stem cell originates, it is likely that the environment in the inflamed, reflux-damaged esophagus mediates the phenotypic switch from a squamous cell to an intestinal-like columnar cell (see **Fig. 1**). This phenotypic switch presumably occurs by altering the expression of a few key master genes that regulate cell phenotype. Candidate master genes that are upregulated in Barrett's esophagus compared with neighboring esophageal squamous epithelium include the transcription factors CDX1, CDX2, and SOX9 (see **Fig. 1**).[21–23] Not only are these genes normally expressed in the intestine but target genes of these transcription factors define an intestinal phenotype.[24,25]

ROLE FOR CDX1, CDX2, AND SOX9 IN BARRETT METAPLASIA

Homeotic genes define the developmental pattern of an organism. Cdx1 and Cdx2 are homeobox genes that specify intestinal epithelial differentiation.[26] Studies in mice suggest that Cdx2 is required for intestinal differentiation and that Cdx1 may specify a columnar cell.[27,28] CDX1 and CDX2 mRNA and protein expression have been detected in esophageal biopsy specimens from nondysplastic Barrett metaplasia, Barrett metaplasia with dysplasia, and Barrett-associated adenocarcinomas, but not in normal esophageal squamous epithelium.[29–31] Sox9 is another transcription factor, expressed by potential stem cells in intestinal crypts, that plays a role in the formation of goblet cells.[32,33] Recently, SOX9 protein has been shown to be expressed in Barrett metaplasia, Barrett with dysplasia, and adenocarcinoma, but not in esophageal squamous epithelium.[23]

HOW GERD MAY INDUCE BARRETT METAPLASIA

Barrett metaplasia is a sequelae of chronic GERD. Components of the refluxed gastric juice (eg, acid, bile salts) and/or the resulting esophageal inflammation (reflux esophagitis) could cause esophageal metaplasia by inducing transcription factors or activating developmental signaling pathways that determine an intestinal phenotype.

Stimulation of the CDX Transcription Factors by GERD

In mouse esophageal squamous epithelial cells, exposure to bile acids or acid activates Cdx2 expression.[34,35] In human esophageal squamous cells (HET1A), exposure to a combination of acid and bile salts increases CDX2 expression and leads to squamous cells forming cryptlike structures and expressing intestinal genes such as Villin, Sucrase-isomaltase, and MUC2[36,37] In addition, data suggest that GERD-induced inflammation activates CDX expression in esophageal squamous epithelial cells. In a rodent model of esophageal intestinal metaplasia, squamous cells begin to express Cdx2 before the development of intestinal metaplasia.[38] In human esophageal biopsies, CDX2 expression has been found in inflamed esophageal squamous epithelium, but not in noninflamed squamous epithelium.[31] In telomerase-immortalized normal esophageal squamous cells established from patients with GERD with and without

Barrett's esophagus, exposure to acid and/or bile salts increased CDX2 expression in the squamous cells from patients with Barrett's esophagus, but not in those from patients with GERD without Barrett's esophagus.[39] Inhibition of nuclear factor-κB (NF-κB), a well-established mediator of GERD-induced inflammation, prevented the increase in CDX2 expression in esophageal squamous cells from patients with Barrett's esophagus in response to acid and/or bile salt exposure, suggesting that inflammatory signaling cascades can also activate CDX2 expression in esophageal squamous cells.[39]

Stimulation of Developmental Signaling Pathways by GERD

An attractive hypothesis is that esophageal activation of developmental signaling pathways involved in maintaining or developing the normal intestine may lead to Barrett metaplasia. These include pathways that are required for normal intestinal development, such as Wnt and Notch, or pathways that are expressed in the embryonic esophagus to maintain a columnar phenotype, such as Hedgehog and Bone Morphogenic Protein (Bmp) 4. Wnt is required to maintain the intestinal crypt progenitor cell population and regulates the expression of Cdx1.[40,41] Wnt pathway activation (as determined by nuclear β-catenin) has not been found in nondysplastic Barrett metaplasia, but has been observed in Barrett metaplasia with dysplasia and in esophageal adenocarcinomas.[42]

The Notch pathway also participates in maintaining the intestinal crypt progenitor pool and perhaps even that of the esophagus.[43] As intestinal cells begin to differentiate, persistent Notch signaling leads to an absorptive enterocyte fate, whereas the lack of Notch signaling leads to a secretory fate as an enteroendocrine, goblet, or Paneth cell.[44,45] Unlike the other developmental signaling pathways, components of the Notch signaling pathway are present in the normal adult esophagus.[46] As noted earlier, CDX2 overexpression in squamous HET1A cells causes the cells to form crypt-like structures.[36] In these same cells, expression of Hes1, a downstream target of Notch, is downregulated by CDX2 overexpression, suggesting that inhibition of Notch signaling by CDX2 may play a role in metaplasia formation.[36] Bile salt exposure has also been shown to decrease expression of Notch pathway components in esophageal adenocarcinoma cells.[47] Recently, in an animal model of reflux and Barrett's esophagus, inhibitors of Notch signaling caused the proliferative Barrett cells to differentiate into goblet cells.[48]

Bmp4 is normally expressed within the stroma of the embryonic columnar-lined esophagus, but it is absent in the adult squamous-lined esophagus.[49,50] In a rodent model of reflux esophagitis and Barrett's esophagus, investigators demonstrated Bmp4 expression in the stroma underlying inflamed esophageal squamous epithelium and specialized intestinal metaplasia, but not in the stroma underlying normal esophageal squamous epithelium.[50] When human esophageal squamous cells were treated with BMP4 in vitro, the squamous cells began to express cytokeratins characteristic of columnar cells, suggesting that stromal BMP4 expression promotes the change in the esophageal epithelium from squamous to columnar.[50]

The Hedgehog signaling pathway likely plays a role in esophageal metaplasia. Sonic hedgehog, the most ubiquitous Hedgehog ligand, is expressed by the embryonic esophagus although it has a columnar epithelium and before it takes on a stratified squamous phenotype.[51] Recently, Sonic hedgehog expression was observed in Barrett metaplasia, but not in normal adult esophageal epithelium.[23] In a mouse model of reflux esophagitis and Barrett's esophagus, Sonic hedgehog expression was found in the Barrett metaplasia as well as in esophageal squamous cells before the development of intestinal metaplasia.[23] Bmp4 is a target of Hedgehog signaling, therefore it was not surprising that stromal BMP4 expression was seen adjacent to Barrett epithelium from esophagectomy specimens.[23] Activation of BMP4 signaling in HET1A cells induced SOX9 expression and subsequent expression of cytokeratins characteristic of columnar cells.[23]

THE MAKING OF BARRETT-ASSOCIATED DYSPLASIA AND ADENOCARCINOMA

The histologic diagnoses of dysplasia and cancer are based on a compilation of morphologic features of the tissue that indicate that the cells have acquired abnormal physiologic properties. In 2000, Hanahan and Weinberg[52] characterized 6 physiologic properties of cancer, also called hallmarks, that normal cells acquire as cancer ensues. These hallmarks include the ability of cells to provide their own growth signals, avoid growth inhibitory signals, resist apoptosis, replicate without limit, synthesize new blood vessels, and invade and metastasize (**Table 1**).[52] Studies have shown that these cancer hallmarks can be acquired by normal cells through disruptions in only a few key growth regulatory pathways including the p16/Retinoblastoma (Rb) and p53 pathways, the Ras signaling pathway, and the telomerase-dependent senescence pathway (see **Table 1**).[53] Recently, cancer-related inflammation has been proposed as a seventh physiologic hallmark of cancer.[54]

KEY GROWTH REGULATORY PATHWAYS THAT CONTRIBUTE TO CARCINOGENESIS
p16/Rb Pathway

To appreciate the contribution of the p16/Rb pathway to carcinogenesis, a brief review of cell proliferation and the cell cycle is presented. The cell cycle encompasses the events that take place for a cell to divide. The cycle is partitioned into 4 phases called gap 1 (G1), DNA synthesis (S), gap 2 (G2), and mitosis (M) (**Fig. 2**). The major point of regulation for cell proliferation occurs in the transition from G1 into S phase of the cell cycle, and Rb is the protein that has master control of this critical juncture (see **Fig. 2**). The ability of cells to bypass this key regulatory point allows them to avoid growth inhibitory signals and to replicate without limit. Although the data are inconclusive, it seems that Rb itself is targeted for inactivation in the later stages of Barrett carcinogenesis (ie, dysplasia and carcinoma), but not in nondysplastic Barrett

Table 1
Cancer hallmarks and the key growth regulatory pathways that contribute to carcinogenesis in Barrett's esophagus

Cancer Hallmark	Key Growth Regulatory Pathway
Provide growth signals	Ras pathway
Avoid growth inhibitory signals	p16/Rb and p53 pathways
Resist apoptosis	p53 pathway, Ras pathway
Replicate without limit	Telomerase-dependent senescence pathway, p16/Rb pathway, p53 pathway
Synthesize new blood vessels	Ras pathway
Invade and metastasize	?? ?? Inflammatory microenvironment
Inflammatory microenvironment	??

The pathways that cause invasion and metastasis and establish the inflammatory microenvironment are not yet known. The establishment of an inflammatory microenvironment might contribute to the ability of tumor cells to invade and metastasize.

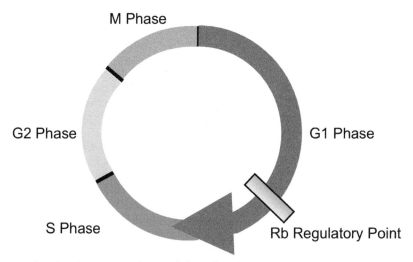

Fig. 2. Cell cycle. There are 4 phases of the cell cycle, gap 1 (G1), DNA synthesis (S), gap2 (G2), and mitosis. The Rb regulatory point controls passage from G1 into S phase.

metaplasia.[55,56] Inactivation of Rb is not the only way to bypass this key regulatory point. p16 is a member of the INK4 family of cell cycle inhibitors. p16 regulates the synthesis of proteins that alter the function of Rb such that cells cannot proceed through the cell cycle. Thus, inactivation of p16 allows cells to pass unhindered from G1 into S phase and is the earliest and most common genetic alteration found in nondysplastic Barrett metplasia.[57] For example, studies have reported p16 inactivation in 73% to 87% of biopsy specimens from patients with nondysplastic Barrett's esophagus.[58,59]

p53 Pathway

p53 is a tumor suppressor gene that inhibits cell proliferation by preventing passage of cells from G1 to S phase of the cell cycle. Like p16, p53 regulates the synthesis of proteins that alter the function of Rb such that cells cannot continue through the cell cycle. p53 also plays a central role in the induction of apoptosis. Therefore, disruption of the p53 pathway gives cells the ability to avoid growth inhibitory signals, to replicate without limit, and to resist apoptosis. Using immunohistochemical staining, mutant p53 expression has been detected in nondysplastic Barrett metaplasia and the frequency of mutant p53 detection increases as dysplasia and adenocarcinoma ensue.[60–62]

Ras Pathway

The Ras pathway is one of the main intracellular signaling cascades activated after the binding of growth factors to their receptors located on the surface of cells.[63] Ras-mediated signals regulate the function of proteins that promote passage from G1 into S phase of the cell cycle and proteins that influence apoptosis.[64] Therefore, disruption of the Ras pathway allows cells to acquire the ability to provide their own growth signals, to resist apoptosis, and to synthesize new blood vessels. Most human tumors demonstrate mutations in Ras (ie, oncogenic Ras) that cause the constant stimulation of downstream signaling cascades independent of growth factor-mediated receptor activation.[65] Expression of oncogenic K-Ras or H-Ras is rare in nonneoplastic Barrett metaplasia; however, expression of both oncogenic Ras proteins has been frequently detected in dysplastic Barrett metaplasia and adenocarcinoma.[66–69] Ras pathway activation does play a role in the early stages of Barrett carcinogenesis; however, it does so in a more physiologic fashion by transmitting signals downstream of the epidermal growth factor receptor (EGFR) and its ligand, transforming growth factor alpha (TGF-α). Increased levels of both EGFR and TGF-α have been found in biopsy samples of nondysplastic Barrett metaplasia and been proposed to account for increased activation of the mitogenic Ras pathway in the early stages of Barrett carcinogenesis.[70]

As discussed earlier, dysfunction of the Ras pathway also allows cells to acquire the ability to synthesize new blood vessels, a process termed angiogenesis. Binding of vascular endothelial growth factors (VEGFs) to their receptors, the vascular endothelial growth factor receptors (VEGFRs) initiates the proliferation and migration of endothelial cells into the tissue via Ras pathway signaling. Nondysplastic Barrett metaplasia has increased expression of VEGF-A, VEGF-C, and VEGFR-2 compared with esophageal squamous epithelium.[71] An enhanced vascular network has been proposed to account for the salmon color characteristic of Barrett's esophagus. Esophageal adenocarcinomas have been shown to express even higher levels of VEGF mRNA and protein compared with nondysplastic or dysplastic Barrett metaplasia.[72]

Telomerase-Dependent Senescence Pathway

Senescence is an intrinsic mechanism of cells that limits their proliferative capacity and is triggered by the progressive loss of telomeres. Telomeres are long stretches of repetitive pieces of DNA located at the ends of chromosomes. With each cell division, some of these telomeric repeats are lost. When telomere loss is such that only a small amount remains, the cell exits the cell cycle into a permanent state of growth arrest, called senescence. To overcome senescence, the cell must maintain telomere length. Telomerase is the enzyme that synthesizes and maintains telomeres.[73] Therefore, disruption of the telomerase-dependent senescence pathway allows cells to replicate without limit and become immortalized. Most normal cells lack telomerase, including normal esophageal squamous cells. Nondysplastic Barrett biopsy specimens express low levels of telomerase, which increase as the degree of dysplasia increases.[74] Esophageal adenocarcinomas also express high levels of telomerase.[75]

Cancer-Related Inflammation

Cancer-related inflammation can be established through 2 pathways: (1) an *extrinsic* pathway in which clinical disorders such as reflux esophagitis cause tissue inflammation that contributes to carcinogenesis, and (2) an *intrinsic* pathway in which the precancerous cells acquire genetic abnormalities that produce an inflammatory tumor microenvironment.[54] The intrinsic and extrinsic inflammatory pathways can converge on certain key downstream targets (eg, cytokines and transcription factors) that promote further inflammation and tumor cell proliferation.[54] Among the key molecules in cancer-related inflammation are transcription factors such as NF-κB and STAT3. NF-κB is well known to mediate both inflammation and tumor progression. NF-κB expression has been found in 40% to 60% of biopsy specimens of Barrett metaplasia and in 61% to 80% of Barrett adenocarcinomas, but in only 13% of biopsy specimens of reflux-injured squamous epithelium.[76,77] Moreover, NF-κB activation has been found to increase as metaplastic Barrett mucosa develops dysplastic changes of progressive severity, suggesting that an inflammatory response might be contributing to carcinogenesis.[77] STAT3 is another transcription factor that is well known to mediate both inflammation and tumorigenesis. In biopsy specimens of Barrett epithelium, expression of the active form of STAT3 increases with the severity of dysplasia, also suggesting a link between the inflammatory response and Barrett carcinogenesis.[78] The molecular mechanisms that mediate invasion and metastasis remain unclear; however, data suggest that perhaps the inflammatory response may be playing a role. For example, matrix metalloproteinases (MMPs) are proteolytic enzymes that can degrade the extracellular matrix and contribute to tumor invasion and metastasis.[79] MMP-1, -2, -7 and -9 expression has been found in nondysplastic Barrett metaplasia and esophageal adenocarcinoma.[80–82] STAT3 has been found to regulate expression of MMP-2 and -9, potentially linking inflammation with Barrett-associated tumor cell invasion and migration.[83]

SUMMARY

The rate of increase in the incidence of esophageal adenocarcinoma in the past several decades is quite startling. GERD and Barrett's esophagus are recognized as major risk factors for esophageal adenocarcinoma. Because most esophageal adenocarcinomas are believed to arise from Barrett's esophagus, the pathogenesis of esophageal metaplasia at the molecular level has become an area of intense investigation. Molecular markers of metaplasia may soon be used to identify individuals at risk for developing Barrett's esophagus rather than relying on epidemiologic risk factors alone. Moreover, the use of molecular markers to identify the stem cell of Barrett's esophagus may allow for the targeting of endoscopic or pharmacologic ablative therapies specifically to the stem cells, thereby eliminating Barrett's esophagus itself and thus the risk for esophageal adenocarcinoma.

Advances in tumor biology have revealed that the complexity of human tumorigenesis can be reduced to disruptions in a few key growth regulatory pathways and an inflammatory microenvironment. This approach provides a useful conceptual basis for evaluating studies on molecular markers for detecting cancer progression and for developing chemoprevention and chemotherapeutic strategies. However, these are pathways comprised of multiple genes and proteins, and pathway disruption can be caused by any number of different modifications in genes and/or in proteins within each pathway. Thus, panels of molecular markers will likely be used to indicate molecular signatures predictive of neoplastic progression, and the molecular characterization of individual tumors will likely be used to tailor therapeutic strategies to an individual patient. Molecular medicine is reshaping our understanding of the biology of Barrett metaplasia, dysplasia, and adenocarcinoma. Clinicians should stay tuned as molecular medicine unfurls endless possibilities to improve the diagnosis and management of patients with Barrett's esophagus.

REFERENCES

1. Jemal A, Thun MJ, Ries LA, et al. Annual report to the nation on the status of cancer, 1975-2005, featuring trends in lung cancer, tobacco use, and tobacco control. J Natl Cancer Inst 2008;100(23):1672–94.
2. Demeester SR. Epidemiology and biology of esophageal cancer. Gastrointest Cancer Res 2009;3(Suppl 2):S2–5.
3. Jemal A, Siegel R, Ward E, et al. Cancer statistics, 2009. CA Cancer J Clin 2009; 59(4):225–49.
4. Wang KK, Sampliner RE. Updated guidelines 2008 for the diagnosis, surveillance and therapy of Barrett's esophagus. Am J Gastroenterol 2008;103(3):788–97.

5. Dulai GS, Guha S, Kahn KL, et al. Preoperative prevalence of Barrett's esophagus in esophageal adenocarcinoma: a systematic review. Gastroenterology 2002; 122(1):26–33.

6. Souza RF. A molecular rationale for the how, when and why of colorectal cancer screening. Aliment Pharmacol Ther 2001;15(4):451–62.

7. Spechler SJ. Clinical practice. Barrett's esophagus. N Engl J Med 2002;346(11): 836–42.

8. Tosh D, Slack JM. How cells change their phenotype. Nat Rev Mol Cell Biol 2002; 3(3):187–94.

9. Guillem PG. How to make a Barrett esophagus: pathophysiology of columnar metaplasia of the esophagus. Dig Dis Sci 2005;50(3):415–24.

10. Johns BA. Developmental changes in the oesophageal epithelium in man. J Anat 1952;86(4):431–42.

11. Yu WY, Slack JM, Tosh D. Conversion of columnar to stratified squamous epithelium in the developing mouse oesophagus. Dev Biol 2005;284(1):157–70.

12. Sawhney RA, Shields HM, Allan CH, et al. Morphological characterization of the squamocolumnar junction of the esophagus in patients with and without Barrett's epithelium. Dig Dis Sci 1996;41(6):1088–98.

13. Sancho E, Batlle E, Clevers H. Signaling pathways in intestinal development and cancer. Annu Rev Cell Dev Biol 2004;20:695–723.

14. Daniely Y, Liao G, Dixon D, et al. Critical role of p63 in the development of a normal esophageal and tracheobronchial epithelium. Am J Physiol Cell Physiol 2004;287(1):C171–81.

15. Glickman JN, Yang A, Shahsafaei A, et al. Expression of p53-related protein p63 in the gastrointestinal tract and in esophageal metaplastic and neoplastic disorders. Hum Pathol 2001;32(11):1157–65.

16. Leedham SJ, Preston SL, McDonald SA, et al. Individual crypt genetic heterogeneity and the origin of metaplastic glandular epithelium in human Barrett's oesophagus. Gut 2008;57(8):1041–8.

17. Colleypriest BJ, Palmer RM, Ward SG, et al. Cdx genes, inflammation and the pathogenesis of Barrett's metaplasia. Trends Mol Med 2009;15(7): 313–22.

18. Epperly MW, Guo H, Shen H, et al. Bone marrow origin of cells with capacity for homing and differentiation to esophageal squamous epithelium. Radiat Res 2004; 162(3):233–40.

19. Sarosi G, Brown G, Jaiswal K, et al. Bone marrow progenitor cells contribute to esophageal regeneration and metaplasia in a rat model of Barrett's esophagus. Dis Esophagus 2008;21(1):43–50.

20. Korbling M, Katz RL, Khanna A, et al. Hepatocytes and epithelial cells of donor origin in recipients of peripheral-blood stem cells. N Engl J Med 2002;346(10): 738–46.

21. Wong NA, Wilding J, Bartlett S, et al. CDX1 is an important molecular mediator of Barrett's metaplasia. Proc Natl Acad Sci U S A 2005;102(21):7565–70.

22. Moons LM, Bax DA, Kuipers EJ, et al. The homeodomain protein CDX2 is an early marker of Barrett's oesophagus. J Clin Pathol 2004;57(10):1063–8.

23. Wang DH, Clemons NJ, Miyashita T, et al. Aberrant epithelial-mesenchymal Hedgehog signaling characterizes Barrett's metaplasia. Gastroenterology 2010; 138(5):1810–22.

24. Chan CW, Wong NA, Liu Y, et al. Gastrointestinal differentiation marker Cytokeratin 20 is regulated by homeobox gene CDX1. Proc Natl Acad Sci U S A 2009; 106(6):1936–41.

25. Traber PG, Wu GD, Wang W. Novel DNA-binding proteins regulate intestine-specific transcription of the sucrase-isomaltase gene. Mol Cell Biol 1992;12(8): 3614–27.
26. Silberg DG, Swain GP, Suh ER, et al. Cdx1 and cdx2 expression during intestinal development. Gastroenterology 2000;119(4):961–71.
27. Gao N, White P, Kaestner KH. Establishment of intestinal identity and epithelial-mesenchymal signaling by Cdx2. Dev Cell 2009;16(4):588–99.
28. Mutoh H, Sakurai S, Satoh K, et al. Cdx1 induced intestinal metaplasia in the transgenic mouse stomach: comparative study with Cdx2 transgenic mice. Gut 2004;53(10):1416–23.
29. Phillips RW, Frierson HF Jr, Moskaluk CA. Cdx2 as a marker of epithelial intestinal differentiation in the esophagus. Am J Surg Pathol 2003;27(11):1442–7.
30. Groisman GM, Amar M, Meir A. Expression of the intestinal marker Cdx2 in the columnar-lined esophagus with and without intestinal (Barrett's) metaplasia. Mod Pathol 2004;17(10):1282–8.
31. Eda A, Osawa H, Satoh K, et al. Aberrant expression of CDX2 in Barrett's epithelium and inflammatory esophageal mucosa. J Gastroenterol 2003;38(1):14–22.
32. Blache P, van de Wetering M, Duluc I, et al. SOX9 is an intestine crypt transcription factor, is regulated by the Wnt pathway, and represses the CDX2 and MUC2 genes. J Cell Biol 2004;166(1):37–47.
33. Bastide P, Darido C, Pannequin J, et al. Sox9 regulates cell proliferation and is required for Paneth cell differentiation in the intestinal epithelium. J Cell Biol 2007;178(4):635–48.
34. Burnat G, Rau T, Elshimi E, et al. Bile acids induce overexpression of homeobox gene CDX-2 and vascular endothelial growth factor (VEGF) in human Barrett's esophageal mucosa and adenocarcinoma cell line. Scand J Gastroenterol 2007;42(12):1460–5.
35. Marchetti M, Caliot E, Pringault E. Chronic acid exposure leads to activation of the cdx2 intestinal homeobox gene in a long-term culture of mouse esophageal keratinocytes. J Cell Sci 2003;116(Pt 8):1429–36.
36. Liu T, Zhang X, So CK, et al. Regulation of Cdx2 expression by promoter methylation, and effects of Cdx2 transfection on morphology and gene expression of human esophageal epithelial cells. Carcinogenesis 2007;28(2):488–96.
37. Hu Y, Jones C, Gellersen O, et al. Pathogenesis of Barrett esophagus: deoxycholic acid up-regulates goblet-specific gene MUC2 in concert with CDX2 in human esophageal cells. Arch Surg 2007;142(6):540–4 [discussion: 544–5].
38. Tatsuta T, Mukaisho K, Sugihara H, et al. Expression of Cdx2 in early GRCL of Barrett's esophagus induced in rats by duodenal reflux. Dig Dis Sci 2005;50(3): 425–31.
39. Huo X, Zhang HY, Zhang XI, et al. Acid and bile salt-induced CDX2 expression differs in esophageal squamous cells from patients with and without Barrett's esophagus. Gastroenterology 2010;139(1):194–203, e1.
40. van de Wetering M, Sancho E, Verweij C, et al. The beta-catenin/TCF-4 complex imposes a crypt progenitor phenotype on colorectal cancer cells. Cell 2002; 111(2):241–50.
41. Lickert H, Domon C, Huls G, et al. Wnt/(beta)-catenin signaling regulates the expression of the homeobox gene Cdx1 in embryonic intestine. Development 2000;127(17):3805–13.
42. Bian YS, Osterheld MC, Bosman FT, et al. Nuclear accumulation of beta-catenin is a common and early event during neoplastic progression of Barrett esophagus. Am J Clin Pathol 2000;114(4):583–90.

43. Fre S, Huyghe M, Mourikis P, et al. Notch signals control the fate of immature progenitor cells in the intestine. Nature 2005;435(7044):964–8.

44. Stanger BZ, Datar R, Murtaugh LC, et al. Direct regulation of intestinal fate by Notch. Proc Natl Acad Sci U S A 2005;102(35):12443–8.

45. van Es JH, van Gijn ME, Riccio O, et al. Notch/gamma-secretase inhibition turns proliferative cells in intestinal crypts and adenomas into goblet cells. Nature 2005;435(7044):959–63.

46. Sander GR, Powell BC. Expression of notch receptors and ligands in the adult gut. J Histochem Cytochem 2004;52(4):509–16.

47. Morrow DJ, Avissar NE, Toia L, et al. Pathogenesis of Barrett's esophagus: bile acids inhibit the Notch signaling pathway with induction of CDX2 gene expression in human esophageal cells. Surgery 2009;146(4):714–21 [discussion: 721–2].

48. Menke V, van Es JH, de Lau W, et al. Conversion of metaplastic Barrett's epithelium into post-mitotic goblet cells by gamma-secretase inhibition. Dis Model Mech 2010;3(1–2):104–10.

49. Que J, Choi M, Ziel JW, et al. Morphogenesis of the trachea and esophagus: current players and new roles for noggin and Bmps. Differentiation 2006;74(7): 422–37.

50. Milano F, van Baal JW, Buttar NS, et al. Bone morphogenetic protein 4 expressed in esophagitis induces a columnar phenotype in esophageal squamous cells. Gastroenterology 2007;132(7):2412–21.

51. Litingtung Y, Lei L, Westphal H, et al. Sonic hedgehog is essential to foregut development. Nat Genet 1998;20(1):58–61.

52. Hanahan D, Weinberg RA. The hallmarks of cancer. Cell 2000;100(1):57–70.

53. Hahn WC, Weinberg RA. Rules for making human tumor cells. N Engl J Med 2002;347(20):1593–603.

54. Colotta F, Allavena P, Sica A, et al. Cancer-related inflammation, the seventh hallmark of cancer: links to genetic instability. Carcinogenesis 2009;30(7): 1073–81.

55. Huang Y, Meltzer SJ, Yin J, et al. Altered messenger RNA and unique mutational profiles of p53 and Rb in human esophageal carcinomas. Cancer Res 1993; 53(8):1889–94.

56. Coppola D, Schreiber RH, Mora L, et al. Significance of Fas and retinoblastoma protein expression during the progression of Barrett's metaplasia to adenocarcinoma. Ann Surg Oncol 1999;6(3):298–304.

57. Klump B, Hsieh CJ, Holzmann K, et al. Hypermethylation of the CDKN2/p16 promoter during neoplastic progression in Barrett's esophagus. Gastroenterology 1998;115(6):1381–6.

58. Wong DJ, Barrett MT, Stoger R, et al. p16INK4a promoter is hypermethylated at a high frequency in esophageal adenocarcinomas. Cancer Res 1997;57(13): 2619–22.

59. Maley CC, Galipeau PC, Li X, et al. The combination of genetic instability and clonal expansion predicts progression to esophageal adenocarcinoma. Cancer Res 2004;64(20):7629–33.

60. Younes M, Lebovitz RM, Lechago LV, et al. p53 protein accumulation in Barrett's metaplasia, dysplasia, and carcinoma: a follow-up study. Gastroenterology 1993; 105(6):1637–42.

61. Hamelin R, Flejou JF, Muzeau F, et al. TP53 gene mutations and p53 protein immunoreactivity in malignant and premalignant Barrett's esophagus. Gastroenterology 1994;107(4):1012–8.

62. Ramel S, Reid BJ, Sanchez CA, et al. Evaluation of p53 protein expression in Barrett's esophagus by two-parameter flow cytometry. Gastroenterology 1992; 102(4 Pt 1):1220–8.

63. Malumbres M, Pellicer A. RAS pathways to cell cycle control and cell transformation. Front Biosci 1998;3:d887–912.

64. Inamdar GS, Madhunapantula SV, Robertson GP. Targeting the MAPK pathway in melanoma: why some approaches succeed and other fail. Biochem Pharmacol 2010;80(5):624–37.

65. Cooper GM. Cellular transforming genes. Science 1982;217(4562):801–6.

66. Meltzer SJ, Mane SM, Wood PK, et al. Activation of c-Ki-ras in human gastrointestinal dysplasias determined by direct sequencing of polymerase chain reaction products. Cancer Res 1990;50(12):3627–30.

67. Lord RV, O'Grady R, Sheehan C, et al. K-ras codon 12 mutations in Barrett's oesophagus and adenocarcinomas of the oesophagus and oesophagogastric junction. J Gastroenterol Hepatol 2000;15(7):730–6.

68. Sommerer F, Vieth M, Markwarth A, et al. Mutations of BRAF and KRAS2 in the development of Barrett's adenocarcinoma. Oncogene 2004;23(2):554–8.

69. Abdelatif OM, Chandler FW, Mills LR, et al. Differential expression of c-myc and H-ras oncogenes in Barrett's epithelium. A study using colorimetric in situ hybridization. Arch Pathol Lab Med 1991;115(9):880–5.

70. Jankowski J, McMenemin R, Hopwood D, et al. Abnormal expression of growth regulatory factors in Barrett's oesophagus. Clin Sci (Lond) 1991;81(5):663–8.

71. Auvinen MI, Sihvo EI, Ruohtula T, et al. Incipient angiogenesis in Barrett's epithelium and lymphangiogenesis in Barrett's adenocarcinoma. J Clin Oncol 2002; 20(13):2971–9.

72. Lord RV, Park JM, Wickramasinghe K, et al. Vascular endothelial growth factor and basic fibroblast growth factor expression in esophageal adenocarcinoma and Barrett esophagus. J Thorac Cardiovasc Surg 2003;125(2):246–53.

73. Shay JW, Bacchetti S. A survey of telomerase activity in human cancer. Eur J Cancer 1997;33(5):787–91.

74. Morales CP, Lee EL, Shay JW. In situ hybridization for the detection of telomerase RNA in the progression from Barrett's esophagus to esophageal adenocarcinoma. Cancer 1998;83(4):652–9.

75. Lord RV, Salonga D, Danenberg KD, et al. Telomerase reverse transcriptase expression is increased early in the Barrett's metaplasia, dysplasia, adenocarcinoma sequence. J Gastrointest Surg 2000;4(2):135–42.

76. Abdel-Latif MM, O'Riordan J, Windle HJ, et al. NF-kappaB activation in esophageal adenocarcinoma: relationship to Barrett's metaplasia, survival, and response to neoadjuvant chemoradiotherapy. Ann Surg 2004;239(4):491–500.

77. O'Riordan JM, Abdel-latif MM, Ravi N, et al. Proinflammatory cytokine and nuclear factor kappa-B expression along the inflammation-metaplasia-dysplasia-adenocarcinoma sequence in the esophagus. Am J Gastroenterol 2005;100(6):1257–64.

78. Dvorak K, Chavarria M, Payne CM, et al. Activation of the interleukin-6/STAT3 anti-apoptotic pathway in esophageal cells by bile acids and low pH: relevance to Barrett's esophagus. Clin Cancer Res 2007;13(18 Pt 1):5305–13.

79. Coussens LM, Fingleton B, Matrisian LM. Matrix metalloproteinase inhibitors and cancer: trials and tribulations. Science 2002;295(5564):2387–92.

80. Herszenyi L, Hritz I, Pregun I, et al. Alterations of glutathione S-transferase and matrix metalloproteinase-9 expressions are early events in esophageal carcinogenesis. World J Gastroenterol 2007;13(5):676–82.

81. Murray GI, Duncan ME, O'Neil P, et al. Matrix metalloproteinase-1 is associated with poor prognosis in oesophageal cancer. J Pathol 1998;185(3):256–61.
82. Salmela MT, Karjalainen-Lindsberg ML, Puolakkainen P, et al. Upregulation and differential expression of matrilysin (MMP-7) and metalloelastase (MMP-12) and their inhibitors TIMP-1 and TIMP-3 in Barrett's oesophageal adenocarcinoma. Br J Cancer 2001;85(3):383–92.
83. Haura EB, Turkson J, Jove R. Mechanisms of disease: insights into the emerging role of signal transducers and activators of transcription in cancer. Nat Clin Pract Oncol 2005;2(6):315–24.

Endoscopic Evaluation and Advanced Imaging of Barrett's Esophagus

Kenneth K. Wang, MD*, Ngozi Okoro, MD,
Ganapathy Prasad, MD, Michel WongKeeSong, MD,
Navtej S. Buttar, MD, Jianmin Tian, MD

KEYWORDS
- Barrett's esophagus • Laser confocal endomicroscopy
- Advanced imaging • Narrow band imaging

ENDOSCOPIC EQUIPMENT: DOES IT MATTER?

Visualization of small mucosal irregularities is becoming increasingly difficult. In the advent of flat adenomas in the colon to subtle lesions in the esophagus and stomach that represent the earliest signs of malignancy, the need to image better has never been more apparent. The 20% miss rate of colonic polyps is undoubtedly related to the inability to view subtle mucosal irregularities. Fortunately, there have been several technical improvements since the fiberoptic endoscope that not only magnify the mucosa but also enhance the resolution of the mucosa so that subtle lesions can be easily visualized.

Resolution is defined in imaging as the ability to resolve 2 small dots adjacent to each other. A high-resolution endoscope could find differences between 2 dots that look like a single dot on standard videoendoscopy. It will be undoubtedly true that there will be even higher-resolution videoendoscopes in the near future.

In the age of high-definition television and its variants, it is important to understand what is meant by the term *resolution* and exactly what it means to endoscopy. Most of the time, high-resolution endoscopy is a term that is used to reference the pixel density of the charge coupled device (CCD) in the endoscope. The CCD is the actual silicon chip that captures light and converts this energy into a digital signal. It is important to recognize that this does not mean that just because you are using a high-resolution

Conflicts of interest: research funding from Olympus Corporation and SpectraScience, and consulting with OncoScope.
Division of Gastroenterology, Mayo Clinic, Rochester, MN, USA
* Corresponding author. Division of Gastroenterology and Hepatology, Mayo Clinic, 200 2nd Street South West, Rochester, MN 55905.
E-mail address: wang.kenneth@mayo.edu

Gastrointest Endoscopy Clin N Am 21 (2011) 39–51
doi:10.1016/j.giec.2010.09.013
1052-5157/11/$ – see front matter © 2011 Elsevier Inc. All rights reserved.

endoscope you are getting a high-resolution image. The visualization will require a high-resolution processor and a video screen that can display high-resolution images. Standard resolution endoscopes were designed to mimic television standards with resolutions of 640 pixel width and 486 lines vertical (National Television System Committee [NTSC] standard in United States, Japan) versus a 576 lines vertical (Phase Alternate Line [PAL] standard in Europe) with pixel densities of approximately 367,000. High-resolution endoscopes that have recently been developed are generally thought of as those with more than 1 million pixels. Current videoendoscopes approach this but most do not exceed 1 million pixels with color chips. The Pentax i-Flex endoscope (Pentax Medical Company, Montvale, NJ, USA) has a 1.25 million pixel CCD, which is what is needed to be able to display in high definition (1280 × 1024 pixels). The current generation Olympus 180 series endoscope (Olympus America Inc, Center Valley, PA, USA) also has 1280 × 1024 resolution and can display in HD mode. However, this does not mean that the endoscopist will see this in HD because the outputs from the EPK-i (Pentax) processor or the Evis Exera II (Olympus) processor include standard video outputs, including Red Green Blue (RGB), Separate Video (S-video or Y/C), composite outputs (NTSC), and HD outputs.

There are differences with endoscopes, most commonly used in the United States, because they all use a so-called color chip. Each pixel of these colored chips is actually created from 3 separate dots, each representing one of the primary colors (red, green, blue), which allows the chip to present a colored image. However, the color chips are generally larger than their monochromatic counterparts and have less resolution. The highest-resolution endoscopes currently available are monochromatic with a color image generated by a color wheel with red, green, and blue filters placed in front of the chip. As the wheel turns, the particular filter in front of the chip is recorded and that image is saved and blended with 2 other images using the other 2 primary colors to create a composite color image. This type of endoscope has not been well received because of the color-streaming effects that are caused when there is water or rapid motion of the endoscope.

ENDOSCOPIC EVALUATION OF BARRETT'S ESOPHAGUS

Barrett's esophagus is an endoscopically defined condition, so its description is critical to the diagnosis of patients suspected of having the condition. Currently, it is the custom to denote the proximal extent of the Barrett's esophagus as well as the maximal circumferential extent in terms of distances from these landmarks to the incisors (**Fig. 1**).

The Barrett's segment is usually described as being salmon colored in appearance and must be distinct from the gastric mucosa, which is also reddish in color. Because the gastroesophageal junction is difficult to endoscopically define, it is typically chosen to be at the level of the tops of the gastric folds, which can be seen in **Fig. 2** where the tops of the folds can be clearly demarcated.

Once the segment length is documented, the next important step is to find any mucosal abnormalities within the mucosal surface. Although there are many different techniques to enhance imaging, it is clear that what is most important is a careful white light examination because most abnormalities can be visualized with a standard endoscope. All mucosal abnormalities should be carefully biopsied. These abnormalities include lesions, such as ulcers, nodules, or just areas of mucosal irregularity (**Figs. 3** and **4**).

Mucosal abnormalities in Barrett's esophagus must be carefully inspected. All mucosal irregularities could contain areas of dysplasia or even frank carcinoma. These

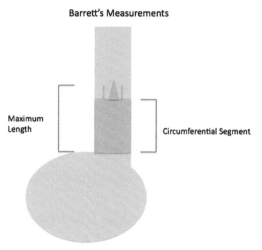

Barrett's Measurements

Maximum
Length

Circumferential Segment

Fig. 1. The current system of classifying the length of Barrett's esophagus. The maximum length and the circumferential segment length should be identified.

abnormal areas, according to recent guidelines, should be individually targeted for histologic sampling. In the setting of Barrett's esophagus with high-grade dysplasia, these abnormalities should undergo mucosal resection because studies have shown that there may be as high as a 40% incidence of carcinoma occurring in these regions.[1] Although white light examination is sufficient to visualize almost all abnormalities, often times there is information that can be obtained using other forms of imaging.

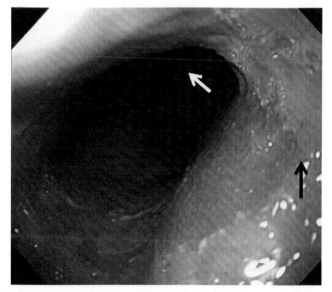

Fig. 2. A typical Barrett's esophagus segment with a proximal squamocolumnar junction at the black arrow and the distal segment at the white arrow at the tops of the gastric folds.

Mucosal Lesions: Classification

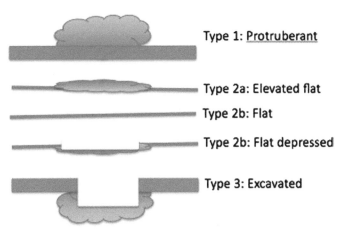

Type 1: <u>Protruberant</u>

Type 2a: Elevated flat

Type 2b: Flat

Type 2b: Flat depressed

Type 3: Excavated

Fig. 3. Classification of lesions. The most common lesions found in Barrett's esophagus are types 2a and 2b, being slightly elevated or flat.

Chromoendoscopy

Chromoendoscopy has also been proposed since the time of fiberoptic endoscopes to enhance imaging. In the esophagus, this was primarily with iodine staining to detect areas of squamous neoplasia. In the case of Barrett's esophagus, most of the effort has been spent on using either a contrast stain (indigo carmine) typically used with

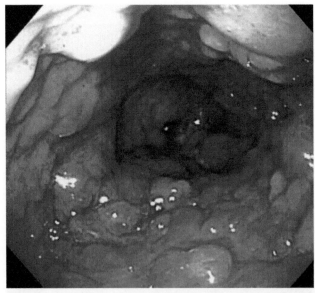

Fig. 4. An example of multiple type 1 lesions that are protuberant into the lumen of the Barrett's esophagus. This example is a polypoid Barrett's esophagus. Each of these polypoid lesions were high-grade dysplasia.

a magnification endoscope (45–200X) to allow visualization of mucosal patterns or an absorptive dye (methylene blue) with an increased uptake that is suggestive of intestinal metaplasia. However, as the area becomes more dysplastic, methylene blue staining decreases (**Fig. 5**).

A recent meta-analysis was performed of 9 studies and 450 subjects that reported on the yield of using methylene blue as a contrast agent for detection of dysplasia compared with random biopsies.[2–9] The variation in the results from the studies was quite remarkable with both markedly positive and negative results. Ultimately, a meta-analysis found that the there was no significant difference between methylene blue and random biopsies in detection of dysplasia.[10] In addition, studies have raised concerns that methylene blue could serve as a photosensitizing agent that might lead to DNA damage when used in Barrett's esophagus.[11] Other agents have been used for chromoendoscopy but there is not sufficient data to draw conclusions regarding their performance.

Narrow Band Imaging

Narrow band imaging (NBI) is a term applied to a specific commercial imaging technique (Olympus America, Center Valley, PA, USA). It involves the use of 2 different wavelengths of filtered light, 415 and 540 nm, for illumination, which is what gives the light a bluish appearance when NBI is activated. The blue illumination, at 414 nm, allows the imaging of the surface capillaries and the green 540 nm illumination allows visualization of vessels at a great depth (**Fig. 6**).

Multiple studies have been published looking at the values of NBI in Barrett's esophagus. In particular, criteria have been established to examine vascular as well as mucosal abnormalities.[12–20] These studies are summarized in **Table 1**.

If one does a meta-analysis on this data, we find that there is a significant advantage in using NBI, particularly in detecting areas of high-grade dysplasia. A pooled sensitivity for the detection of high-grade dysplasia on a per patient basis is 0.88 with a 95% confidence interval of 79% to 93%. It is important to point out that this advantage has been established with a high-resolution endoscope that is not commercially available in the United States. The GIF Q240Z and Q260Z (Olympus America, Center

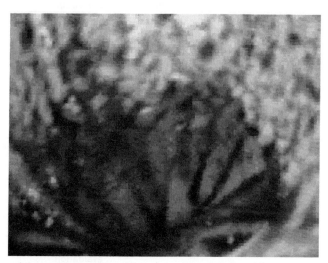

Fig. 5. Image of the gastroesophageal junction with methylene blue staining. The areas of nonstaining could be dysplastic tissue or inflammatory non-Barrett's mucosa.

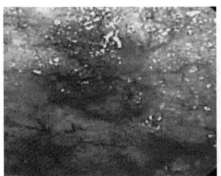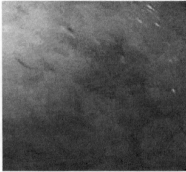

Fig. 6. Images of NBI of an erythematous patch seen below and then under NBI above. The borders are clearer and mucosal detail is easier to appreciate.

Valley, PA, USA) are high-resolution endoscopes primarily used in Asia and Europe and are not approved by the US Food and Drug Administration (FDA). There is some data to suggest that the GIF 180 series endoscope that is used in the United States is of benefit with NBI, but this benefit has only been found in one study that compared the GIF 180 (Olympus America, Center Valley, PA, USA) series to a low-resolution endoscope.[21] This makes it more difficult to discern whether this improvement in dysplasia detection is caused by increased resolution or NBI. In addition, these studies have been done in enriched populations with high proportions of subjects with high-grade dysplasia. The pooled specificity is probably not relevant to most practices because of this skewed population.

Table 1
Studies of NBI values in Barrett's esophagus

Authors	Mean Age (y)	Patients (n)	Total Lesions Examined	Study Design	Endoscope Type
Kara et al[14–16] 2006	65.0	63	161	Cross-sectional Post hoc image evaluation	GIF Q240Z
Kara et al[14–16] 2006	66.0	20	47	Cross-sectional Real-time evaluation	GIF Q240Z
Sharma et al[18] 2006	64.0	51	204	Cross-sectional Image evaluation	GIF Q240Z
Curvers et al[17] 2008	67.0	84	165	Cross-sectional Real-time evaluation	GIF Q240Z
Singh et al[12] 2009	61.9	109	1021	Cross-sectional Post hoc image evaluation	GIF Q240Z
Goda et al[19] 2007	60.0	58	217	Cross-sectional Real-time evaluation	GIF Q240Z
Anagnostopoulos et al[34] 2007	62.1	50	344	Cross-sectional Real-time evaluation	GIF Q240Z
Kara et al[13] 2005	66.0	28	36	RCT, Real-time evaluation	GIF Q260Z

Abbreviation: RCT, randomized controlled trial.

There are other modalities that can enhance the appearance of blood vessels although these rely on postprocessing techniques. The Fuji Intelligent Chromo Endoscopy (FICE) system (Fujinon, Wayne, NJ, USA) uses a white light source and processes the color obtained through spectral analysis, which is obtained from a CCD and a prism mounted on the tip of the endoscope. The light from the endoscope always appears white, unlike the blue-green light seen from the Olympus system. The FICE system is selectable for different enhancement modes that can be optimized for a specific function. There are only small series using FICE for detection of Barrett's esophagus.[22] The other system is I-Scan from Pentax (Montvale, NJ, USA), which offers 3 levels of postprocessing enhancements to emphasize the contrast, surface, and tone in addition to standard white light examination. These enhancements use the high-definition image to emphasize features, such as color, contrast, or the short wavelengths of light reflected from the surface. These enhancements have been used to increase visualization of mucosal breaks in the esophagus.[23]

Magnification Techniques

Several magnification techniques have been developed to enhance the imaging in Barrett's esophagus. It should be recognized that standard endoscopes have magnified the image from the esophagus by several fold depending on the size of the viewing monitor, which has made it much easier to appreciate mucosal detail. A variation on the standard endoscope is the endocytoscope, which can be placed on a standard endoscope processor and has a powerful magnifying lens that focuses on the CCD. The endocytoscope is designed to fit through a therapeutic endoscope (outside diameter of 3.4 mm) to allow magnification of suspicious areas. The degree of magnification achieved can either be 450 X or 1100 X depending on the instrument used. To visualize the mucosa, a topical contrast agent, such as indigo carmine or methylene blue, must be applied because high magnification without contrast agents does not allow any imaging. These contrast agents allow for visualization of glandular structures (**Fig. 7**).

Endocytoscopy has been used to define areas of dysplasia within Barrett's esophagus, but initial results have not been promising primarily because of difficulties with maintaining a stable image.[24] Because of the high magnification, any motion distorts the image such as that caused by patients' heartbeat and esophageal motility. Nonetheless, this entity can be useful in determining areas of cancer and dysplasia in controlled situations.[25]

Magnification endoscopes have a 200-fold magnification capability. There is a trade-off with these magnifying endoscopes; generally, the higher the magnification the shorter the focal length of imaging, meaning that the scopes become impractical to use at anything but a targeted lesion. In addition, the endoscopes tend to be of larger diameter, which makes them less tolerable in the upper gastrointestinal tract. Magnification endoscopy has been used in conjunction with chromoendoscopy for more than a decade in Barrett's esophagus.[26–34] As with most imaging modalities, there is a problem with inter-observer agreement (k <0.4) because there is difficulty in identifying mucosa types that are glandular in nature, such as between Barrett's esophagus and gastric-cardia type of tissue.[33] In addition, there is a suggestion that in prospective studies, magnification endoscopy does not enhance detection of intestinal metaplasia.[32]

Confocal Laser Endomicroscopy and Optical Coherence Tomography

Confocal laser endomicroscopy (CLE) and optical coherence tomography (OCT) have similar principles. Both are able to focus laser light to a specific plane deep to the surface and to magnify the appearance of microscopic structures approximately

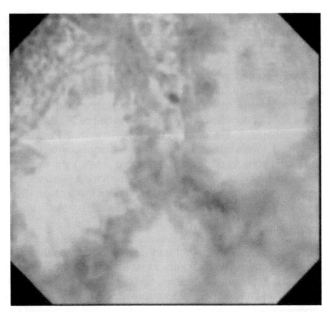

Fig. 7. Endocytoscopy of Barrett's crypts on endoscopy with methylene blue contrast. The crypts are regular in appearance.

400 X. Both use light interference as the basis for their effect. In CLE, this focusing is done using a pinhole that focuses the laser light entering the pinhole to light from a specific depth. With optical coherence tomography, there is a reference light path that is used to create interference patterns with the reflected light from the surface. Adjustments in the reference path length have the effect of increase penetration into the mucosa. OCT yields an image similar to B-mode ultrasound with good resolution of layer structure; whereas, CLE offers more of a tangential imaging of the surface glandular structure. Both of these techniques allow better imaging with lateral resolution potential of approximately 10 μ.[35] By giving an intravenous injection of 10% sodium fluorescein, the mucosa can be seen with CLE after 2 to 3 minutes. This contrast enables the confocal laser microscope to view the intravascular space where there are leaks in the capillary membranes and actually see areas of extravasation of dye into the extravascular space. However, this type of imaging does not allow direct visualization of cells and their structure, but only the shadow of the cells that is cast because one is able to image the surrounding parenchyma because of the vascular structures present. Overall, when a disorganized pattern is seen in both the capillaries and the mucosal structure, there is reasonable certainty that there is dysplasia present **(Fig. 8)**.

The reported sensitivity of an endoscope-based system of CLE is 92.9% and a specificity of 98.4% for detection of neoplasia in Barrett's esophagus in a cohort study of 63 subjects.[36] This system takes advantage of the confocal principles by having a zoom feature that can focus from 0μ to 250 μ from the surface, which allows the user to scan down the length of a gland. Because the LCE obtains views parallel to the surface rather than the perpendicular, as achieved with standard histology, this zoom may be important when trying to differentiate dysplastic lesions. The resolution of this system is also superior to the probe system (0.7 μ vs 1.0 μ for the probe systems) and has a wider field of view (500 μ vs 240 μ). However, the endoscope system is

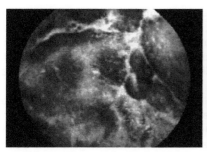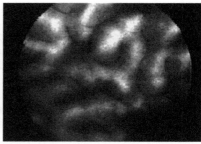

Fig. 8. Confocal laser images. The first is of irregular glandular structure in Barrett's esophagus with high-grade dysplasia; whereas, the bottom is of benign typical gastric mucosal glands.

integrated into an endoscope with a diameter of 12.8 mm and the confocal system acquires images continuously at 0.8-second intervals, which leads to a large number of unusable images.

The probe system has also been reported to be approximately 75% sensitive and 90% specific for detection of dysplasia in a small cohort study (n = 38) with 2 endoscopists.[37] This probe system is more convenient to apply because the site that is being optically investigated can be visualized with the endoscope. With the integrated endoscope system, the site being imaged is out of view during the imaging and must be estimated from the distance from a suction mark deliberately made by the endoscopist. An advantage of the dedicated endoscope is reusability; whereas, the probe can only be used 20 times with some degradation of the imaging during reuse. The likelihood that these systems may decrease biopsies is suggested by a recent randomized controlled study with the dedicated endoscope system, which indicated that with the system much more dysplasia can be detected and excluded in other patients.[38] These are promising devices that may supplant or supplement histology in the near future. However, implementation into clinical practice will be dependent on the demonstration that these tools will actually improve patient outcomes in patients with dysplasia or cancer.

Spectroscopy-Based Diagnostic Tools

These tools include devices that can analyze light that is typically scattered or that undergo fluorescence from the mucosal surface. Spectroscopy does not actually give an image; it gives a quantitative assessment of the light that is reflected from the mucosal surface. This assessment can be made on the intensity of the light that is captured or by the amount of light that is detected over a period of time. Both of these methods can give specific information about the tissue type. By using careful analysis of the spectroscopic patterns, an estimate can be made regarding the optical characteristics of the mucosa. This estimate can include nuclear size, crowding, degree of vascularity, and the organization of the intestinal glands. These technologies would incorporate the interpretation of the information into the device rather than require image interpretation by a physician. These are all point technologies that cannot examine an entire area but only potentially suspicious regions.

One of the first spectroscopic technologies was laser-induced fluorescence, which can measure fluorescence from naturally occurring fluorophores, such as flavin adenine dinucleotide (FADH), nicotinamide adenine dinucleotide (NAD), tryptophan, and collagen. Porphyrins are blood breakdown products that also form a large portion of the fluorescent peak. By analysis of the degree of autofluorescence, the determination of neoplasia can be made. Generally, areas with decreased autofluorescence have an increased propensity toward neoplasia. Excitation-emission matrices of areas of cell cultures of keratinocytes and squamous carcinoma cells are shown in **Fig. 9**. It is clear that even in vivo, there are distinct differences in the autofluorescence pattern between benign and malignant cell lines.

Laser-induced fluorescence has been found to detect dysplasia in Barrett's esophagus and has actually been approved by the FDA for use in colon polyps for adenoma detection.[39,40] However, this technology has not been commercialized at this point.

Diffuse reflectance spectroscopy, which examines light scattering from the surface of the mucosa, has also been found to differentiate normal from neoplastic tissues throughout the gastrointestinal tract.[41,42] This technology is based on the increased scattering of light from cells that are less organized and have greater-sized nuclei. There have been refinements on examination of this light spectra, the most notable being low-coherence enhanced back scattering, which has been used to focus on short light path scattering phenomenon, allowing the detection of nanoscale changes in cells.[43] This low-coherence enhanced back scattering uses nonlinear optics in its derivations, which means that the degree of resolution is not limited by the wavelength of light. This practice can theoretically resolve nanoscale-type changes in the mucosa.[44] These changes in tissue characteristics have been applied to the duodenum to detect field effects of pancreatic cancer and to the distal colon for the field effects of more proximal colon neoplasia.[45,46] This method would allow identification of patients at risk of carcinoma simply by applying a probe to a more conveniently available structure. For instance, assessment of the buccal mucosa could be used to determine whether or not there is neoplastic risk in the lungs or in the esophagus. Although this is intriguing, it is clear that there is a need for large-scale clinical trials to demonstrate the ability of these technologies to function in the clinical situation.

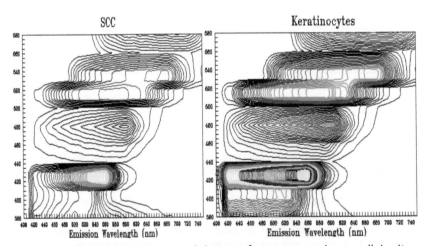

Fig. 9. Two autofluorescence spectroscopic images of squamous carcinoma cells in vitro and keratinocytes. They were examined using a multitude of excitation laser wavelengths and plotted against the fluorescence seen. The colors of the lines indicate the intensity of the light. As can be seen, normal keratinocytes have much greater intrinsic fluorescence than cancer cell lines, which is what is typically found.

SUMMARY

Enhanced visualization techniques are available for Barrett's esophagus and have promise in the detection of dysplasia and cancer. Several of these techniques, such as narrow band imaging and chromoendoscopy, are being applied clinically. These techniques will allow the endoscopist to screen the surface of the Barrett's esophagus to detect areas of neoplasia. Once detected, it is hoped that either magnification techniques, such as confocal laser endomicroscopy, or spectroscopic techniques can be of value in allowing in vivo real-time diagnostic capabilities.

ACKNOWLEDGMENTS

The authors wish to acknowledge the support of the National Cancer Institute R01CA097048, R01CA111603, and R21CA122426 and the Mayo Foundation.

REFERENCES

1. Nijhawan PK, Wang KK. Endoscopic mucosal resection for lesions with endoscopic features suggestive of malignancy and high-grade dysplasia within Barrett's esophagus. comment. Gastrointest Endosc 2000;52:328–32.
2. Canto MI, Setrakian S, Willis J, et al. Methylene blue-directed biopsies improve detection of intestinal metaplasia and dysplasia in Barrett's esophagus. Gastrointest Endosc 2000;51:560–8.
3. Canto MI, Setrakian S, Willis JE, et al. Methylene blue staining of dysplastic and nondysplastic Barrett's esophagus: an in vivo and ex vivo study. Endoscopy 2001;33:391–400.
4. Sharma P, Topalovski M, Mayo MS, et al. Methylene blue chromoendoscopy for detection of short-segment Barrett's esophagus. Gastrointest Endosc 2001;54:289–93.
5. Wo JM, Ray MB, Mayfield-Stokes S, et al. Comparison of methylene blue-directed biopsies and conventional biopsies in the detection of intestinal metaplasia and dysplasia in Barrett's esophagus: a preliminary study. Gastrointest Endosc 2001;54:294–301.
6. Gossner L, Pech O, May A, et al. Comparison of methylene blue-directed biopsies and four-quadrant biopsies in the detection of high-grade intraepithelial neoplasia and early cancer in Barrett's oesophagus. Dig Liver Dis 2006;38:724–9.
7. Lim CH, Rotimi O, Dexter SP, et al. Randomized crossover study that used methylene blue or random 4-quadrant biopsy for the diagnosis of dysplasia in Barrett's esophagus [see comment]. Gastrointest Endosc 2006;64:195–9.
8. Horwhat JD, Maydonovitch CL, Ramos F, et al. A randomized comparison of methylene blue-directed biopsy versus conventional four-quadrant biopsy for the detection of intestinal metaplasia and dysplasia in patients with long-segment Barrett's esophagus. Am J Gastroenterol 2008;103:546–54.
9. Ormeci N, Savas B, Coban S, et al. The usefulness of chromoendoscopy with methylene blue in Barrett's metaplasia and early esophageal carcinoma. Surg Endosc 2008;22:693–700.
10. Ngamruengphong S, Sharma VK, Das A. Diagnostic yield of methylene blue chromoendoscopy for detecting specialized intestinal metaplasia and dysplasia in Barrett's esophagus: a meta-analysis. Gastrointest Endosc 2009;69:1021–8.
11. Olliver JR, Wild CP, Sahay P, et al. Chromoendoscopy with methylene blue and associated DNA damage in Barrett's oesophagus. Lancet 2003;362:373–4.

12. Singh R, Karageorgiou H, Owen V, et al. Comparison of high-resolution magnification narrow-band imaging and white-light endoscopy in the prediction of histology in Barrett's oesophagus. Scand J Gastroenterol 2009;44:85–92.
13. Kara MA, Peters FP, Rosmolen WD, et al. High-resolution endoscopy plus chromoendoscopy or narrow-band imaging in Barrett's esophagus: a prospective randomized crossover study. Endoscopy 2005;37:929–36.
14. Kara MA, Bergman JJ, Kara MA, et al. Autofluorescence imaging and narrow-band imaging for the detection of early neoplasia in patients with Barrett's esophagus. Endoscopy 2006;38:627–31.
15. Kara MA, Ennahachi M, Fockens P, et al. Detection and classification of the mucosal and vascular patterns (mucosal morphology) in Barrett's esophagus by using narrow band imaging. Gastrointest Endosc 2006;64:155–66.
16. Kara MA, Peters FP, Fockens P, et al. Endoscopic video-autofluorescence imaging followed by narrow band imaging for detecting early neoplasia in Barrett's esophagus [see comment]. Gastrointest Endosc 2006;64:176–85.
17. Curvers W, Baak L, Kiesslich R, et al. Chromoendoscopy and narrow-band imaging compared with high-resolution magnification endoscopy in Barrett's esophagus [see comment]. Gastroenterology 2008;134:670–9.
18. Sharma P, Marcon N, Wani S, et al. Non-biopsy detection of intestinal metaplasia and dysplasia in Barrett's esophagus: a prospective multicenter study. Endoscopy 2006;38:1206–12.
19. Goda K, Tajiri H, Ikegami M, et al. Usefulness of magnifying endoscopy with narrow band imaging for the detection of specialized intestinal metaplasia in columnar-lined esophagus and Barrett's adenocarcinoma [see comment]. Gastrointest Endosc 2007;65:36–46.
20. Anagnostopoulos GK, Yao K, Kaye P, et al. Magnification endoscopy with Narrow Band Imaging in Barrett's esophagus. J Clin Gastroenterol 2006;40:S192–3.
21. Wolfsen HC, Crook JE, Krishna M, et al. Prospective, controlled tandem endoscopy study of narrow band imaging for dysplasia detection in Barrett's Esophagus [see comment]. Gastroenterology 2008;135:24–31.
22. Osawa H, Yamamoto H, Yamada N, et al. Diagnosis of endoscopic Barrett's esophagus by transnasal flexible spectral imaging color enhancement. J Gastroenterol 2009;44:1125–32.
23. Hoffman A, Basting N, Goetz M, et al. High-definition endoscopy with i-Scan and Lugol's solution for more precise detection of mucosal breaks in patients with reflux symptoms. Endoscopy 2009;41:107–12.
24. Pohl H, Koch M, Khalifa A, et al. Evaluation of endocytoscopy in the surveillance of patients with Barrett's esophagus [see comment]. Endoscopy 2007;39:492–6.
25. Tomizawa Y, Abdulla HM, Prasad GA, et al. Endocytoscopy in esophageal cancer. Gastrointest Endosc Clin N Am 2009;19:273–81.
26. Guelrud M, Herrera I, Essenfeld H, et al. Enhanced magnification endoscopy: a new technique to identify specialized intestinal metaplasia in Barrett's esophagus. Gastrointest Endosc 2001;53:559–65.
27. Connor MJ, Sharma P. Chromoendoscopy and magnification endoscopy in Barrett's esophagus [review]. Gastrointest Endosc Clin N Am 2003;13:269–77.
28. Kiesslich R, Mergener K, Naumann C, et al. Value of chromoendoscopy and magnification endoscopy in the evaluation of duodenal abnormalities: a prospective, randomized comparison. Endoscopy 2003;35:559–63.
29. Meining A, Rosch T, Kiesslich R, et al. Inter- and intra-observer variability of magnification chromoendoscopy for detecting specialized intestinal metaplasia at the gastroesophageal junction. Endoscopy 2004;36:160–4.

30. Toyoda H, Rubio C, Befrits R, et al. Detection of intestinal metaplasia in distal esophagus and esophagogastric junction by enhanced-magnification endoscopy. Gastrointest Endosc 2004;59:15–21.
31. Rey JF, Inoue H, Guelrud M. Magnification endoscopy with acetic acid for Barrett's esophagus. Endoscopy 2005;37:583–6.
32. Ferguson DD, DeVault KR, Krishna M, et al. Enhanced magnification-directed biopsies do not increase the detection of intestinal metaplasia in patients with GERD. Am J Gastroenterol 2006;101:1611–6.
33. Mayinger B, Oezturk Y, Stolte M, et al. Evaluation of sensitivity and inter- and intra-observer variability in the detection of intestinal metaplasia and dysplasia in Barrett's esophagus with enhanced magnification endoscopy [see comment]. Scand J Gastroenterol 2006;41:349–56.
34. Anagnostopoulos GK, Yao K, Kaye P, et al. Novel endoscopic observation in Barrett's oesophagus using high resolution magnification endoscopy and narrow band imaging. Aliment Pharmacol Ther 2007;26:501–7.
35. Testoni P-A, Mangiavillano B. Optical coherence tomography in detection of dysplasia and cancer of the gastrointestinal tract and bilio-pancreatic ductal system. World J Gastroenterol 2008;14:6444–52.
36. Kiesslich R, Gossner L, Goetz M, et al. In vivo histology of Barrett's esophagus and associated neoplasia by confocal laser endomicroscopy. Clin Gastroenterol Hepatol 2006;4:979–87.
37. Pohl H, Rosch T, Vieth M, et al. Miniprobe confocal laser microscopy for the detection of invisible neoplasia in patients with Barrett's oesophagus. Gut 2008; 57:1648–53.
38. Dunbar KB, Okolo P 3rd, Montgomery E, et al. Confocal laser endomicroscopy in Barrett's esophagus and endoscopically inapparent Barrett's neoplasia: a prospective, randomized, double-blind, controlled, crossover trial. Gastrointest Endosc 2009;70:645–54.
39. Wang KK, Densmore J. Laser induced fluorescence in the diagnosis of esophageal carcinoma. In: Lambert R, editor. Proceeding of the European SPIE. Amsterdam: Elsevier; 1995. p. 132–4.
40. von Holstein CS, Nilsson AM, Andersson-Engels S, et al. Detection of adenocarcinoma in Barrett's oesophagus by means of laser induced fluorescence. Gut 1996;39:711–6.
41. Georgakoudi I, Van DJ. Characterization of dysplastic tissue morphology and biochemistry in Barrett's esophagus using diffuse reflectance and light scattering spectroscopy [review]. Gastrointest Endosc Clin N Am 2003;13:297–308.
42. Badizadegan K, Backman V, Boone CW, et al. Spectroscopic diagnosis and imaging of invisible pre-cancer. Faraday Discuss 2004;126:265–79 [discussion: 303–11].
43. Kim YL, Liu Y, Wali RK, et al. Low-coherent backscattering spectroscopy for tissue characterization. Appl Opt 2005;44:366–77.
44. Kim YL, Turzhitsky VM, Liu Y, et al. Low-coherence enhanced backscattering: review of principles and applications for colon cancer screening. J Biomed Opt 2006;11:041125.
45. Liu Y, Brand RE, Turzhitsky V, et al. Optical markers in duodenal mucosa predict the presence of pancreatic cancer [see comment]. Clin Cancer Res 2007;13: 4392–9.
46. Roy HK, Turzhitsky V, Kim Y, et al. Association between rectal optical signatures and colonic neoplasia: potential applications for screening. Cancer Res 2009;69: 4476–83.

Staging of Early Adenocarcinoma in Barrett's Esophagus

Tom C.J. Seerden, MD, PhD[a], Alberto Larghi, MD, PhD[b],*

KEYWORDS

• Barrett's esophagus • Early cancer • Staging

In the last decade, endoscopic mucosal resection (EMR) with or without ablative therapy has emerged as the standard treatment alternative to surgical resection for the management of high-grade intraepithelial neoplasia (HGIN) and mucosal adenocarcinoma arising in the context of Barrett's esophagus (BE).[1-4] Endoscopic treatment has an excellent 5-year survival, with the advantages of a low rate of complications, better quality of life, and a negligible procedure-related mortality rate, as compared with surgery.[3,5] The basis for endoscopic treatment is the extremely low risk, if any, of lymph node metastasis (LNM) for both HGIN and early cancers confined to the mucosal layer.[6,7] On the other hand, the risk of LNM increases exponentially up to 50% when the tumor infiltrates in the deepest layers of the submucosa, rendering surgical treatment mandatory.[7,8]

The shift of the therapeutic approach to early BE cancer toward local endoscopic and ablative therapies has dramatically increased the importance of pretherapeutic staging, to precisely estimate the depth of tumor infiltration and to exclude LNM in order to identify those patients who will benefit the most from local endoscopic therapy. The crucial question that needs to be answered is: "Is the tumor invasion restricted to the mucosal layer?" This question can be correctly answered by using a staging strategy that combines careful endoscopic inspection of the lesion, endoscopic ultrasonography (EUS), and mucosectomy used as a staging procedure. In the this article, the authors discuss the different staging modalities to assess early adenocarcinoma in BE and propose a systematic staging strategy that will help to differentiate patients who are eligible for endoscopic therapy from those who require surgery with or without neoadjuvant chemotherapy as a primary treatment.

The authors have nothing to disclose.
a Department of Gastroenterology, Amphia Hospital, Molengracht 21, 4818 CK, Breda, The Netherlands
b Digestive Endoscopy Unit, Department of Surgery, Università Cattolica del Sacro Cuore, Largo Agostino Gemelli 8, 00168 Rome, Italy
* Corresponding author.
E-mail address: albertolarghi@yahoo.it

Gastrointest Endoscopy Clin N Am 21 (2011) 53–66
doi:10.1016/j.giec.2010.09.006
1052-5157/11/$ – see front matter © 2011 Elsevier Inc. All rights reserved.

RISK OF LYMPH NODE METASTASIS IN EARLY ADENOCARCINOMA IN BE

Differently from all other hollow viscus organs of the gastrointestinal (GI) tract, the esophagus is characterized by the presence of lymphatic vessels starting from the lamina propria and the muscularis mucosae. Mucosal and submucosal lymphatics form a complex interconnecting network of vessels that intermittently pierce the muscularis propria, draining into regional lymph nodes and, in some patients, directly into the thoracic duct. This lymphatic anatomy allows early and widespread dissemination of esophageal carcinoma and probably also contributes to skipping lymph nodes in esophageal cancers.[9]

The most important risk factor predicting LNM in both early adenocarcinoma and squamous cell (SCC) esophageal cancers is the depth of infiltration of the lesion.[7,10] In early esophageal cancers and more in general in all early cancers of the GI tract,[11] the risk of LNM can be better defined by dividing the mucosal (m) and submucosal (sm) layers into 3 sections: T1m1 (epithelium),T1m2 (lamina propria), and T1m3 (muscularis mucosae); and T1sm1 (upper third), T1sm2 (middle third), and T1sm3 (lower third) (**Fig. 1A**). In BE, because of the existence of a newly formed muscularis mucosae just beneath the Barrett's epithelium,[12] the mucosal layer is divided in 4 sections: T1m1 (epithelium), T1m2 (newly formed muscularis mucosae), T1m3 (lamina propria), and T1m4 (original muscularis mucosae) (see **Fig. 1B**).

The prevalence of LNM in early adenocarcinoma in BE limited to the mucosal layer varies from 0% to 4%.[3,7,13–17] This range of reported LNM reflects the small number of subjects included in some of the published studies. A more realistic estimation of less than 1% is obtained when a pooled analysis of all the data is performed.[18] Thus, early adenocarcinoma seems to behave less aggressively than SCC, where the risk of LNM starts to increase with invasion of the muscularis mucosa (m3).[18] This less aggressive pattern of lymph node spreading of esophageal adenocarcinoma is also seen in the first third of the submucosal layer (T1sm1), where recent studies have suggested a much lower risk of lymph node involvement (0%–8%)[15,19] as compared with T1sm1 SCC (7%–53%)[14,20–22] and to adenocarcinoma infiltrating the lower two-thirds of the submucosa (T1sm2-3)[15,19] (26%–67%). Because of these features, some investigators have suggested that endoscopic treatment should also be considered for patients with adenocarcinoma and superficial low-risk submucosal invasion, even though this view is still a matter of debate.[23] The discrepancy of LNM between SCC

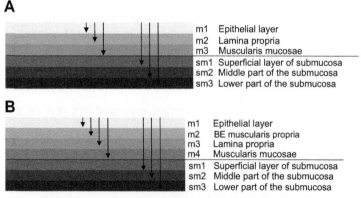

A

m1 Epithelial layer
m2 Lamina propria
m3 Muscularis mucosae
sm1 Superficial layer of submucosa
sm2 Middle part of the submucosa
sm3 Lower part of the submucosa

B

m1 Epithelial layer
m2 BE muscularis propria
m3 Lamina propria
m4 Muscularis mucosae
sm1 Superficial layer of submucosa
sm2 Middle part of the submucosa
sm3 Lower part of the submucosa

Fig. 1. (*A*) T1 subclassification in normal esophagus. (*B*) T1 subclassification in Barrett's esophagus.

and adenocarcinoma in BE has been explained in part as a result of the chronic inflammatory insult to the esophagus by the long-lasting reflux and of the repetitive bouts of esophagitis in patients with BE, which can both cause occlusion of lymphatic channels and hamper early tumor cell spread along the extensive submucosal lymphatic network.[14]

ENDOSCOPIC STAGING OF EARLY ADENOCARCINOMA IN BE

Staging of patients with HGIN and early Barrett's cancer referred for endoscopic therapy starts with a careful endoscopic inspection of the Barrett's epithelium. Recent studies showed that up to 80% of subjects referred for workup of HGIN and early Barrett's cancer without visible lesions will have at least 1 visible abnormality detected.[24,25] This remarkable discrepancy illustrates that in clinical practice, endoscopists still do not pay enough attention to carefully inspect the BE for visible lesions and thereby already go wrong with the first step of staging: look and correctly identify macroscopically your early Barrett's cancers. Most experts, therefore, recommend the use of high-resolution endoscopes (with or without magnification), because they provide superior imaging quality. The addition of chromoendoscopy with staining agents, such as methylene blue, indigo carmine, and acetic acid, or the use of virtual chromoendoscopy, such as the one obtained with narrow-band imaging and Fujinon Intelligent Chromo Endoscopy (FICE; Fujinon Inc, Saitama, Japan), may further increase the endoscopist capability of recognizing subtle mucosal lesions.[24,26–29]

Another important key point in the endoscopic evaluation of patients with BE and early cancer is the search for synchronous lesions that can occur in up to 30% of T1m cancers.[30] One of the most common mistakes made is to concentrate too much on one visible lesion and overlook other areas. This mistake can lead to biopsies being taken too soon and bleeding obscuring other areas of malignancy. Whether a dry biopsy technique with the spraying of diluted epinephrine would help to avoid this problem and lead to higher detection of early cancers and multifocal carcinoma needs to be studied in the near future.[31] It is conceivable that a thorough inspection and 4-quadrant biopsy mapping in long-segment Barrett can be facilitated by this technique and result in less false-negative biopsies and missed macroscopic occult neoplastic lesions.

Once the early cancer is clearly detected, the macroscopic appearance of the lesion should then be carefully evaluated. Recent studies from both the Wiesbaden and the Amsterdam groups have shown that the macroscopic type of early cancers classified according to the Paris classification (**Fig. 2**) helps to predict the depth of tumor infiltration and thus the potential risk for LNM.[11,32–34] According to this classification, which is adopted from the Japanese Gastric Cancer Association classification of early gastric cancer,[35] superficial lesions are classified as type 0 and divided as follows: polypoid or protruding (type 0-I), slightly elevated (type 0-IIa), completely flat (type 0-IIb), slightly depressed (0-II c), excavated (type 0-III), or a combination of types (for example, type 0-IIa-b implies that the tumor has elevated and flat parts and type 0-IIa-c implies that the tumor has elevated and depressed parts). The 2 aforementioned studies demonstrated that in approximately 85% of the cases, early superficial neoplastic lesions in BE are type II lesions (**Table 1**). Type 0-IIb lesions, which are harder to detect compared with other types, were found to have infiltration limited to the mucosa and a good grade of differentiation in up to 96% of the cases. These characteristics make these lesions more suitable for endoscopic resection because there is a low probability for LNM. The rate of submucosal infiltration seems to be slightly higher for type 0-IIa lesions and mixed types as compared with type 0-IIb lesions,

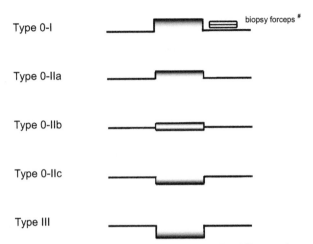

Fig. 2. Paris classification of superficial neoplastic lesions. #The difference between type II and the other types can be made if the lesion is more elevated or depressed as closed biopsy forceps.

but lower than type 0-I and 0-IIc lesions in which invasion of the submucosa occurs in about one-fourth of the cases (see **Table 1**). On the other hand, type 0-III lesions have a much higher rate of submucosal infiltration, which is usually deep, making these lesions not suitable for endoscopic treatment.

The importance of endoscopic staging using high-resolution endoscopes is well documented by a study by May and colleagues,[32] in which 100 subjects with early esophageal cancer (81 with adenocarcinoma in BE, and 19 with SCC) underwent staging with both high-resolution endoscopy (HRE) and high-resolution endosonography using high-frequency mini probes (HFP). The endoscopic and ultrasonographic staging procedures showed a similar diagnostic accuracy (82.9% vs 79.6%), which increased to 84% when the two procedures were combined. HRE and HFP provided a high level of diagnostic accuracy for mucosal and submucosal tumours located in the tubular part of the oesophagus. With submucosal tumours located at the oesophagogastric junction or with infiltration of the first third of the submucosa, however, the diagnostic meaningfulness of both techniques felt significantly.[32] Of note, conventional radial EUS that was also performed as part of the staging workup, correctly staged suspicious lymph nodes in 15 of the 16 subjects who underwent surgical resection, with a sensitivity and specificity in predicting N1 status of 100% and 92%, respectively.

Table 1
Summary of the largest published series that have examined the relationship between macroscopic appearance of early cancer in BE and the degree of infiltration

Macroscopic Appearance of Early Cancer Lesions[11]						
Authors	0-I	0-IIa	0-IIb	0-IIc	0-IIa-IIb	0-IIa-IIc
Pech et al[33]	42/47 (89%)	115/134 (86%)	82/85 (96%)	12/16 (75%)	—	51/62 (82%)
Peters et al[34]	17/23 (74%)	31/34 (91%)	11/11 (100%)	3/4 (75%)	12/13 (92%)	57/63 (90%)

The information in parentheses indicates the rate of subjects with infiltration confined to the mucosal layer at histology compared with total number of subjects.

These results again suggest that assessment of the macroscopic type of the superficial neoplastic lesions by experienced endoscopists helps to predict submucosal infiltration and is at least as accurate as HFP without, however, the chance to perform an adequate lymph node staging.

ENDOSCOPIC ULTRASOUND STAGING

Endoscopic ultrasonography in the staging of early esophageal carcinoma in BE is performed for 2 main purposes: to differentiate between mucosal (T1m) and submucosal (T1sm) tumors and to exclude deeper invasion in the muscle layer and rule out the presence of LNM. Two types of endosonographic instruments have been used to address these issues in the staging of early adenocarcinoma in BE. The first option is to use the conventional echo-endoscope scanner (7.5 –12.0 MHz) that displays the esophageal wall as a 5-layer structure and has good penetration in depth, which allows for good visualization of the structures beyond the esophageal wall in the search for the presence of suspicious lymph nodes. The second option is to use high-frequency miniprobes, which work at higher frequencies (15–30 MHz). These probes are advanced in the esophageal lumen through the working channel of a normal endoscope with the possibility of placing the probe under endoscopic view in close contact with the lesion to be examined. The high frequencies available with the HFP, result in a finer resolution of the esophageal wall that is seen as consisting of 9 different layers. The first 4 layers are the mucosa; the first and second layer is the epithelium, the third hyperechoic layer is the lamina propria, and the fourth hypoechoic layer is the muscularis mucosae. The fifth layer is the submucosa, which is thin and appears hyperechoic. The muscularis propria consists of 2 hypoechoic layers (inner circular muscle layer and outer longitudinal muscle layer) separated by a thin hyperechoic layer. The ninth hyperechoic layer corresponds to the adventitia. The higher resolution of the esophageal wall with the use of the HFP is obtained at the expense of the penetration depth with loss in accuracy for the evaluation of surrounding lymph nodes.

Major limitations of conventional echo-endoscopes in performing a proper T staging of early adenocarcinoma in BE have been pointed out in different studies. Most early cancers in BE are small and achieving a proper positioning with this scope can be cumbersome, if not impossible.[36] In a recent series from the Wiesbaden group, conventional radial echo-endoscope could not visualize the target lesion in 33% of the subjects and T stage was correctly assessed in only 49% of the cohort. The oblique optical view of linear, and some radial, EUS models renders accurate positioning of the echo-endoscope at the level of the early neoplasia difficult. Moreover, once inflated, the balloon can compress the lesion making identification and accurate staging sometimes impossible. Another disadvantage of conventional echo-endoscopes is that the muscularis mucosa cannot be visualized separately and therefore accurate differentiation between mucosal versus submucosal invasion is difficult. Submucosal tumors are suspected when the third hyperechogenic layer corresponding with the submucosa is narrowed or if a hypoechogenic disruption of the interface between the second and third layer is observed.[37,38] Overall, conventional EUS tends to overstage early esophageal cancers, a phenomenon that occurs in 10% to 28% of the patients with T1 lesions.[36,39–42] Falk and colleagues[42] attributed the tendency to overstage to the accompanying reflux esophagitis (which made differentiation between mucosal and submucosal difficult), to artifacts caused by overlapping folds pulled up by the balloon, and to tangential imaging. This inclination to overstage because of the difficultly in the discrimination between mucosal and submucosal invasion appears to also exist for deep submucosal tumors (sm3), which, in a recent study, have been classified as T2 in about 65% of the cases.[41] Unlike mucosal and submucosal lesions, however, in this case overstaging has no impact on patient management.

Although conventional EUS appears to be inadequate for T staging of early Barrett's cancer, standard endosonographic evaluation can reveal unsuspected malignant lymphadenopathy in these patients.[36,43] In a recent article, Shami and colleagues[43] reported that conventional endosonography detected suspicious adenopathy in 7 out of 25 subjects with HGIN and early cancer referred for endoscopic management. EUS-guided fine needle aspiration (EUS-FNA) confirmed malignancy in 5 of these 7 subjects, resulting in change of management in 20% of the entire cohort.[43] Pech and colleagues[44] reported the presence of lymph nodes in 45 out of 100 subjects with early BE cancer. A total of 36 had paraesophageal lymph nodes in the tumor area smaller than 1 cm or larger than 1 cm in another area (category 2); whereas, in 9 subjects, highly suspicious lymph nodes were seen (category 3). In contrast to the study of Shami and colleagues, they did not perform EUS-FNA. Overall, LNM was found in 2 of the 3 subjects without lymphadenopathy on EUS who underwent surgery because of submucosal invasion and in all of the 6 subjects with highly suspicious lymph nodes and submucosal invasion who also underwent surgery. Subjects with category 2 lymph nodes were followed up and no one showed progression of the adenopathy; approximately one-third of the subjects showed regression. Overall, sensitivity, specificity, and positive and negative predictive values of EUS evaluation without performance of the FNA for lymph node staging were 75%, 97%, 75%, and 98%, respectively.[44] Because several reports have demonstrated that compared with EUS, EUS-FNA improved sensitivity, specificity, and accuracy of preoperative lymph node staging, it seems appropriate to perform EUS-FNA of suspected malignant lymph node whenever feasible without passing the primary tumor to maximize staging accuracy.[45,46]

Confronted with the poor accuracy of conventional EUS for T staging, several groups have investigated whether the additional use of HFP could be of value in this clinical setting (**Fig. 3**).[18] In **Table 2**, the results of the studies published on the performance of HFP in subjects with BE and HGIN and early cancer are summarized.[18] Diagnostic accuracy ranged from 73.5% to 95.0%, in part reflecting the small number of subjects evaluated in earlier studies and the inclusion of early SCC in the cohort of subjects evaluated.

A more realistic idea of the performance of these probes comes from the analysis of the 2 largest studies published up to now that included 94 and 106 subjects.[32,47] Both studies reached similar conclusions: (1) the performance of HFP is significantly better for lesions localized in the tubular esophagus (mostly SCC lesions) than those at the EGJ, where the large majority of cancers in BE develop; and (2) the performance of HFP in assessing infiltration of the submucosa is poor, especially for lesions localized at the EGJ. In the article by Chemaly and colleagues,[47] 70% of the subjects with submucosal invasion at HFP were found to have a mucosal tumor at histologic analysis of the EMR or surgical specimen. This finding means that a large number of subjects would have been incorrectly referred to surgery based on the HFP findings. In the article by May and colleagues,[32] the overall sensitivity of HFP for submucosal infiltration was only 48%, which decreased to 14.3% for EGJ tumors. The poor results obtained were mainly caused by a difficulty in recognizing tumors with only initial infiltration of the upper third layer of the submucosa (sm1); while tumors infiltrating the second and third submucosal layers (sm2–sm3) were correctly diagnosed in most of the cases. Recognition of deep submucosal invasion, however, can also be accomplished with conventional EUS.

Several reasons are being proposed to explain the rather mediocre accuracy of HFP in BE.[7,32,42,47,48] Firstly, tissue architecture of columnar epithelium differs from the layered architecture in squamous mucosa, which makes a clear transmission

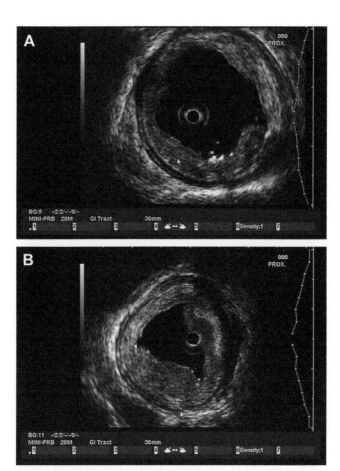

Fig. 3. (*A*) HFP ultrasonography of T1m1 adenocarcinoma in Barrett's esophagus. (*B*) HFP ultrasonography of T1sm1 adenocarcinoma in Barrett's esophagus.

between wall layers more difficult.[38] In addition, concomitant inflammatory changes in the esophageal mucosa, which are also often seen in patients taking proton pump inhibitors with reflux-induced BE, can make correct assessment of tumor infiltration difficult. Secondly and more importantly, adequate water preparation filling of the esophageal lumen while performing the HFP examination in the distal esophagus is often hard to successfully accomplish and to maintain for an adequate period of time to complete the examination. The main reasons for this difficulty are the extremely high motility of the distal esophageal segment and the presence of a hiatal hernia, which is common in patients with BE. The use of balloon-sheathed catheters has been attempted but without substantial advantages over the use of conventional HFP.[47,49] Because of the overall poor performance, the use of the HFP in the evaluation of early BE tumors has been discouraged, even by the group that has published most of the articles on this topic.[50] The only rule for these probes that can still be considered is the evaluation of tumors in the tubular esophagus when under certain conditions a combination of endoscopic resection and photodynamic therapy/thermal ablation is contemplated.[50]

In summary, studies examining the role of EUS in Barrett's adenocarcinoma have shown that conventional EUS and HFP alone are insufficient to accurately assess the

Table 2
Accuracy of HFP in early esophageal cancer

Authors	n	Histologic T1a/T1b	Sensitivity for T1a (%)	Specificity for T1a (%)	Accuracy (%)
Scotiniotis et al[37]	22	17/5	100.0	94.0	95.0
Buskens et al[7]	45	24/21	79.0	95.0	87.0
Larghi et al[6]	48	35/13	—	—	85.0
Esaki et al[49]	40	30/10	100.0/50.0	82.0/87.5	78.0/59.0
Chemaly et al[47]	102	81/21	62.0	76.5	73.5
Rampado et al[48]	55	30/25	63.3	88.0	75.0
Pech et al[44]	55	44/11	89.0	27.0	76.0
May et al[32]	94	69/25	91.2	48.0	79.6

depth of tumor infiltration and, in particular, to rule out early submucosal invasion. On the other hand, exclusion of suspicious lymph nodes with conventional EUS followed by FNA, if necessary, still play a central role in the pretherapeutic staging of these patients.

ENDOSCOPIC RESECTION AND HISTOLOGY

The frequent incongruent results of conventional EUS and HFP with the pathologic staging of Barrett's adenocarcinoma[42,51,52] provided by the specimens obtained by EMR has led several investigators to examine the role of this therapeutic procedure as a staging modality.[6,34,42,53] The aim of EMR staging is to acquire an objective, histologic T staging of the resected lesion with the possibility of evaluating other prognostic factors, such as the degree of tumor differentiation, invasion of lymphatic vessels (L status), and veins (V status),[53,54] which cannot be assessed with any of the other staging modalities described previously. On the resected specimen, the pathologist can accurately determine whether the tumor has breached the muscularis mucosa and entered into the submucosa, thus overcoming the difficulty in assessing this fundamental parameter by EUS and HFP. Staging EMR offers the unique possibility of obtaining all the information needed to base the final treatment decision on.[5,47] In this sense, EMR specimen should be seen first as a diagnostic/staging procedure, recovering its initial meaning when it was first introduced in Japan under the name of strip-off biopsy to increase the probability of diagnosing gastric cancer in subjects with intestinal metaplasia,[55] and then as a treatment procedure.

The availability of the entire lesion with EMR allows a better diagnostic accuracy than biopsy specimens obtained by standard biopsy forceps.[56] Discrepancies in the diagnosis between biopsy samples and EMR specimens have been shown to be more prevalent when lesions are larger than 1 cm and when a less extensive biopsy sampling is performed before EMR.[57] Peters and colleagues[34] reported that the histologic diagnosis of focal lesions before EMR changed after histologic evaluation of the resection specimen in 49% of cases, which led to a relevant change in treatment decision in 30% of the subjects.

The precise histopathologic subclassification shown in **Fig. 1**A, B, however, cannot be used to characterize invasion depth in the EMR specimen that does not contain the full thickness of the submucosa. Classifying submucosal penetration depth in EMR specimens based on the estimated relative penetration into the submucosa (sm1, sm2, and sm3) proved to be inaccurate.[34] Instead, a quantitative micrometric measure in microns of the depth of submucosal invasion from the bottom of the muscularis mucosae can be performed. As reported in a large series from the Amsterdam group, 2 cancers were initially classified as sm2 cancers; whereas, an exact measurement showed a submucosal penetration depth of only 120 μm and 200 μm.[34] The explanation that the investigators proposed for this inaccuracy is that only a part of the submucosa is available for evaluation in EMR specimens and, therefore, an accurate subdivision into 3 equal parts (sm1–3) is impossible to make. Although measurement of submucosal penetration depth may also have some limitations because of (1) flattening of the submucosa by pinning the specimens down after the resection, (2) artifacts caused by the submucosal lifting before ER, and (3) the artificial shrinkage caused by the fixation process, these investigators strongly thought that measurement of the submucosal infiltration depth in micrometers is more reliable than an sm1 to 3 classification for early Barrett's neoplasia.

Other limitations of the EMR specimen include the assessment of the freedom from tumor of the lateral and the basal margins of the specimen (R status), which is important to establish the therapeutic efficacy of the EMR procedure. Coagulation artifacts that occur in up to 25% of the cases can make evaluation of the completeness of the resection of the lateral margins difficult, if not impossible,[34] and tangential orientation of the specimen on the slides can render evaluation of the exact depth of cancer penetration impossible. To limit the tangential orientation of specimens, it is important to adequately stretch and pin down the specimen immediately after its retrieval, before fixation in formalin. Given this significant possibility of relevant artifacts, histologic evaluation of EMR specimens should be performed by a pathologist with experience in this field.

Results from studies reporting the histologic evaluation of EMR specimens from a large cohort of subjects with early BE neoplasia demonstrated that most early cancers in this clinical setting are well to moderately differentiated (G1–G2)[34,58] whereas, poorly differentiated (G3) cancers are rare (7.5%). Moreover, G1 differentiated tumors rarely have lymphatic or vascular invasion and in the majority (93%–94%) of cases are confined to the mucosal layer.[34,58] On the other hand, G2 to G3 cancers invaded the submucosa more frequently (27%–40%), with lymphatic and vascular invasion found almost exclusively in submucosal tumors.[34,58]

In summary, EMR represents the most accurate staging procedure to assess depth of infiltration of the tumor and offers vital information to decide the optimal treatment for patients with early BE cancers. If EMR specimen shows submucosal invasion, patients should be referred for evaluation of the feasibility of surgical resection; whereas, patients with mucosal cancers can be managed endoscopically with the diagnostic endoscopic resection also serving as the first step in their endoscopic treatment. For patients with additional lesions and for those with positive resection margins, further treatment is still possible after EMR, including a repeat EMR procedure with or without ablative therapy or, if not possible, surgical resection.

ADDITIONAL STAGING MODALITIES

In the staging of advanced esophageal cancer, computed tomography (CT) and positron emission tomography (PET) have been reported to be of value to exclude distant and lymph node metastases.[59] However, in early esophageal cancers, adequate differentiation between T1 and greater than T1 stages is not possible with CT. If EUS and EMR have revealed a T1m neoplasm, the risk for distant metastasis is not relevant, making CT and PET unnecessary. If submucosal invasion is encountered, staging should also focus on locoregional invasion and distant metastasis. Some prefer to follow a staging protocol as in advanced esophageal cancer, including EUS, ultrasound study of the neck, and CT scanning of thorax and abdomen.[60] Other think that CT scan has no influence on tumor-node-metastasis (TNM) classification if conventional EUS is part of staging.[44]

To the authors' best knowledge there are no studies performed to evaluate the role of PET scan in early BE cancers. Based on the results of studies in subjects with more advanced esophageal cancer,[59,61] the authors strongly believe that routine PET should not be performed for staging early BE cancers. Arguments against the use of PET scan are the same arguments that limit the usefulness of CT (ie, the absence of distant metastasis in these patients and the fact that complete EUS evaluation is almost always possible because of the nonobstructive nature of early tumors). A comparative study with EUS and PET in more advanced esophageal cancers has also demonstrated that the addition of PET to complete EUS staging did not alter locoregional and celiac lymph node staging.[62]

PROPOSED STAGING STRATEGY

The main goal of the staging of patients with early BE neoplasia is to identify patients who are eligible for endoscopic therapy and differentiate them from those who require surgical management. To make the correct patient selection, a combined staging strategy and a systematic approach are necessary (**Box 1**), which consists of

---

Box 1
Proposed staging approach for early adenocarcinoma in Barrett's esophagus

Endoscopy

1. Systematically inspect Barrett's esophagus with high-resolution endoscopes with chromoendoscopy (real or virtual).
2. Identify any mucosal abnormalities.
3. Classify any observed lesions according to the Paris classification.
4. Search for additional synchronous lesions because of the multifocal nature of early BE cancer.
5. Perform target biopsies of any mucosal abnormalities followed by 4 quadrant biopsy.

EUS

1. Exclude invasion of the muscularis propria.
2. Evaluate the presence of suspicious lymph nodes and distant metastases.
3. Perform EUS-FNA of suspected lymph nodes and distant metastasis whenever possible.

Endoscopic resection and histology

1. Perform an endoscopic resection of any endoscopically visible lesions that lift up after submucosal injection.
2. Perform a histologic evaluation of the resected specimen for depth of infiltration, tumor differentiation, lymphatic vessels and vein infiltration, and tumor infiltration of resection margins.
3. Select the treatment based on histologic evaluation of the EMR specimen.

CT and PET scan

1. There is a debatable role in the setting of early BE cancers.

endoscopy evaluation, EUS, and EMR. The staging should always start with a systematic, careful inspection of Barrett's epithelium using high-resolution endoscopes and chromoendoscopy (real or virtual). Suspected areas should be carefully inspected and neoplastic lesions should be identified and classified according to the Paris classification before biopsies are performed. In the case of type II-b lesions, the risk for submucosal invasion is low and EMR should then be considered as the next step in the staging protocol, without the need to exclude LNM with EUS. If other types of lesions (type Ia–b, IIa–IIc, III) are encountered, the authors think that conventional EUS still has a role to exclude deep submucosal and greater than T1 invasion, but more importantly to rule out the presence of locoregional lymph nodes and eventually of distant metastasis. When suspicious lymph nodes are seen, EUS-FNA should be performed whenever is possible. If there are no contraindications for endoscopic resection and there is no definitive cytologic diagnosis of LNM, early neoplasms in BE need to be removed by EMR, performed as a final staging procedure. Pathologic examination of the resection specimen must evaluate invasion depth, resection margins, tumor differentiation, and vascular and lymph vessel infiltration. Based on these findings, the final decision on which is the most appropriate treatment option for evaluated patients can be precisely made.

ACKNOWLEDGMENTS

The authors thank Dr Oliver Pech and the Wiesbaden group for the pictures of high-frequency probe evaluation in patients with early adenocarcinoma in BE.

REFERENCES

1. Gossner L. The role of endoscopic resection and ablation therapy for early lesions. Best Pract Res Clin Gastroenterol 2006;20:867–76.
2. Pech O, Ell C. Endoscopic therapy of Barrett's esophagus. Curr Opin Gastroenterol 2009;25:405–11.
3. Pech O, Behrens A, May A, et al. Long-term results and risk factor analysis for recurrence after curative endoscopic therapy in 349 patients with high-grade intraepithelial neoplasia and mucosal adenocarcinoma in Barrett's oesophagus. Gut 2008;57:1200–6.
4. Ginsberg GG. Endoscopic approaches to Barrett's oesophagus with high-grade dysplasia/early mucosal cancer. Best Pract Res Clin Gastroenterol 2008;22: 751–72.
5. Pech O, May A, Rabenstein T, et al. Endoscopic resection of early oesophageal cancer. Gut 2007;56:1625–34.
6. Larghi A, Lightdale CJ, Memeo L, et al. EUS followed by EMR for staging of high-grade dysplasia and early cancer in Barrett's esophagus. Gastrointest Endosc 2005;62:16–23.
7. Buskens CJ, Westerterp M, Lagarde SM, et al. Prediction of appropriateness of local endoscopic treatment for high-grade dysplasia and early adenocarcinoma by EUS and histopathologic features. Gastrointest Endosc 2004;60:703–10.
8. Feith M, Stein HJ, Siewert JR. Pattern of lymphatic spread of Barrett's cancer. World J Surg 2003;27:1052–7.
9. Rice TW. Superficial oesophageal carcinoma: is there a need for three-field lymphadenectomy? Lancet 1999;354:792–4.
10. Pennathur A, Farkas A, Krasinskas AM, et al. Esophagectomy for T1 esophageal cancer: outcomes in 100 patients and implications for endoscopic therapy. Ann Thorac Surg 2009;87:1048–54.

11. The Paris endoscopic classification of superficial neoplastic lesions: esophagus, stomach, and colon. Gastrointest Endosc 2003;58:S3–43.

12. Takubo K, Sasajima K, Yamashita K, et al. Double muscularis mucosae in Barrett's esophagus. Hum Pathol 1991;22:1158–61.

13. Ell C, May A, Pech O, et al. Curative endoscopic resection of early esophageal adenocarcinomas (Barrett's cancer). Gastrointest Endosc 2007;65: 3–10.

14. Stein HJ, Feith M, Bruecher BL, et al. Early esophageal cancer: pattern of lymphatic spread and prognostic factors for long-term survival after surgical resection. Ann Surg 2005;242:566–73.

15. Westerterp M, Koppert LB, Buskens CJ, et al. Outcome of surgical treatment for early adenocarcinoma of the esophagus or gastro-esophageal junction. Virchows Arch 2005;446:497–504.

16. Rice TW, Blackstone EH, Goldblum JR, et al. Superficial adenocarcinoma of the esophagus. J Thorac Cardiovasc Surg 2001;122:1077–90.

17. Bollschweiler E, Baldus SE, Schroder W, et al. High rate of lymph-node metastasis in submucosal esophageal squamous-cell carcinomas and adenocarcinomas. Endoscopy 2006;38:149–56.

18. Pech O, Gunter E, Ell C. Endosonography of high-grade intra-epithelial neoplasia/early cancer. Best Pract Res Clin Gastroenterol 2009;23:639–47.

19. Liu L, Hofstetter WL, Rashid A, et al. Significance of the depth of tumor invasion and lymph node metastasis in superficially invasive (T1) esophageal adenocarcinoma. Am J Surg Pathol 2005;29:1079–85.

20. Eguchi T, Nakanishi Y, Shimoda T, et al. Histopathological criteria for additional treatment after endoscopic mucosal resection for esophageal cancer: analysis of 464 surgically resected cases. Mod Pathol 2006;19:475–80.

21. Tachibana M, Hirahara N, Kinugasa S, et al. Clinicopathologic features of superficial esophageal cancer: results of consecutive 100 patients. Ann Surg Oncol 2008;15:104–16.

22. Kim DU, Lee JH, Min BH, et al. Risk factors of lymph node metastasis in T1 esophageal squamous cell carcinoma. J Gastroenterol Hepatol 2008;23: 619–25.

23. Manner H, May A, Pech O, et al. Early Barrett's carcinoma with "low-risk" submucosal invasion: long-term results of endoscopic resection with a curative intent. Am J Gastroenterol 2008;103:2589–97.

24. Kara MA, Smits ME, Rosmolen WD, et al. A randomized crossover study comparing light-induced fluorescence endoscopy with standard videoendoscopy for the detection of early neoplasia in Barrett's esophagus. Gastrointest Endosc 2005;61:671–8.

25. Kara MA, Peters FP, Rosmolen WD, et al. High-resolution endoscopy plus chromoendoscopy or narrow-band imaging in Barrett's esophagus: a prospective randomized crossover study. Endoscopy 2005;37:929–36.

26. Osawa H, Yamamoto H, Yamada N, et al. Diagnosis of endoscopic Barrett's esophagus by transnasal flexible spectral imaging color enhancement. J Gastroenterol 2009;44:1125–32.

27. Wolfsen HC, Crook JE, Krishna M, et al. Prospective, controlled tandem endoscopy study of narrow band imaging for dysplasia detection in Barrett's esophagus. Gastroenterology 2008;135:24–31.

28. Canto MI. Acetic-acid chromoendoscopy for Barrett's esophagus: the "pros". Gastrointest Endosc 2006;64:13–6.

29. Pohl J, May A, Rabenstein T, et al. Comparison of computed virtual chromoendoscopy and conventional chromoendoscopy with acetic acid for detection of neoplasia in Barrett's esophagus. Endoscopy 2007;39:594–8.

30. Altorki NK, Lee PC, Liss Y, et al. Multifocal neoplasia and nodal metastases in T1 esophageal carcinoma: implications for endoscopic treatment. Ann Surg 2008; 247:434–9.

31. Pohl J, Nguyen-Tat M, Manner H, et al. "Dry biopsies" with spraying of dilute epinephrine optimize biopsy mapping of long segment Barrett's esophagus. Endoscopy 2008;40:883–7.

32. May A, Gunter E, Roth F, et al. Accuracy of staging in early oesophageal cancer using high resolution endoscopy and high resolution endosonography: a comparative, prospective, and blinded trial. Gut 2004;53:634–40.

33. Pech O, Gossner L, Manner H, et al. Prospective evaluation of the macroscopic types and location of early Barrett's neoplasia in 380 lesions. Endoscopy 2007;39: 588–93.

34. Peters FP, Brakenhoff KP, Curvers WL, et al. Histologic evaluation of resection specimens obtained at 293 endoscopic resections in Barrett's esophagus. Gastrointest Endosc 2008;67:604–9.

35. Japanese Gastric Cancer Association. Japanese classification of gastric carcinoma–2nd English edition–response assessment of chemotherapy and radiotherapy for gastric carcinoma: clinical criteria. Gastric Cancer 2001;4:1–8.

36. Pech O, Gunter E, Dusemund F, et al. Value of high-frequency miniprobes and conventional radial endoscopic ultrasound in the staging of early Barrett's carcinoma. Endoscopy 2010;42:98–103.

37. Scotiniotis IA, Kochman ML, Lewis JD, et al. Accuracy of EUS in the evaluation of Barrett's esophagus and high-grade dysplasia or intramucosal carcinoma. Gastrointest Endosc 2001;54:689–96.

38. Bergman JJ. The endoscopic diagnosis and staging of oesophageal adenocarcinoma. Best Pract Res Clin Gastroenterol 2006;20:843–66.

39. Zuccaro G Jr, Rice TW, Vargo JJ, et al. Endoscopic ultrasound errors in esophageal cancer. Am J Gastroenterol 2005;100:601–6.

40. Kutup A, Link BC, Schurr PG, et al. Quality control of endoscopic ultrasound in preoperative staging of esophageal cancer. Endoscopy 2007;39:715–9.

41. Pech O, Gunter E, Dusemund F, et al. Accuracy of endoscopic ultrasound in preoperative staging of esophageal cancer: results from a referral center for early esophageal cancer. Endoscopy 2010;42:456–61.

42. Falk GW, Catalano MF, Sivak MV, et al. Endosonography in the evaluation of patients with Barrett's esophagus and high-grade dysplasia. Gastrointest Endosc 1994;40:207–12.

43. Shami VM, Villaverde A, Stearns L, et al. Clinical impact of conventional endosonography and endoscopic ultrasound-guided fine-needle aspiration in the assessment of patients with Barrett's esophagus and high grade dysplasia or intramucosal carcinoma who have been referred for endoscopic ablation therapy. Endoscopy 2006;38:157–61.

44. Pech O, May A, Gunter E, et al. The impact of endoscopic ultrasound and computed tomography on the TNM staging of early cancer in Barrett's esophagus. Am J Gastroenterol 2006;101:2223–9.

45. Vazquez-Sequeiros E, Norton ID, Clain JE, et al. Impact of EUS-guided fine-needle aspiration on lymph node staging in patients with esophageal carcinoma. Gastrointest Endosc 2001;53:751–7.

46. Brijbassie A, Shami VM. Esophageal cancer: ultrasonography. Gastroenterol Clin North Am 2009;38:93–104, viii.
47. Chemaly M, Scalone O, Durivage G, et al. Miniprobe EUS in the pretherapeutic assessment of early esophageal neoplasia. Endoscopy 2008;40:2–6.
48. Rampado S, Bocus P, Battaglia G, et al. Endoscopic ultrasound: accuracy in staging superficial carcinomas of the esophagus. Ann Thorac Surg 2008;85: 251–6.
49. Esaki M, Matsumoto T, Moriyama T, et al. Probe EUS for the diagnosis of invasion depth in superficial esophageal cancer: a comparison between a jelly-filled method and a water-filled balloon method. Gastrointest Endosc 2006;63:389–95.
50. May A. Stop confusing us with EUS prior to endoscopic resection. Endoscopy 2008;40:71–2.
51. Conio M, Repici A, Cestari R, et al. Endoscopic mucosal resection for high-grade dysplasia and intramucosal carcinoma in Barrett's esophagus: an Italian experience. World J Gastroenterol 2005;11:6650–5.
52. Waxman I, Raju GS, Critchlow J, et al. High-frequency probe ultrasonography has limited accuracy for detecting invasive adenocarcinoma in patients with Barrett's esophagus and high-grade dysplasia or intramucosal carcinoma: a case series. Am J Gastroenterol 2006;101:1773–9.
53. Odze RD, Lauwers GY. Histopathology of Barrett's esophagus after ablation and endoscopic mucosal resection therapy. Endoscopy 2008;40:1008–15.
54. Stolte M, Kirtil T, Oellig F, et al. The pattern of invasion of early carcinomas in Barrett's esophagus is dependent on the depth of infiltration. Pathol Res Pract 2010;206:300–4.
55. Tada M, Karita M, Yanai H, et al. [Endoscopic therapy of early gastric cancer by strip biopsy]. Gan To Kagaku Ryoho 1988;15:1460–5 [in Japanese].
56. Mino-Kenudson M, Hull MJ, Brown I, et al. EMR for Barrett's esophagus-related superficial neoplasms offers better diagnostic reproducibility than mucosal biopsy. Gastrointest Endosc 2007;66:660–6.
57. Hull MJ, Mino-Kenudson M, Nishioka NS, et al. Endoscopic mucosal resection: an improved diagnostic procedure for early gastroesophageal epithelial neoplasms. Am J Surg Pathol 2006;30:114–8.
58. Vieth M, Ell C, Gossner L, et al. Histological analysis of endoscopic resection specimens from 326 patients with Barrett's esophagus and early neoplasia. Endoscopy 2004;36:776–81.
59. van Vliet EP, Heijenbrok-Kal MH, Hunink MG, et al. Staging investigations for oesophageal cancer: a meta-analysis. Br J Cancer 2008;98:547–57.
60. Curvers WL, Bansal A, Sharma P, et al. Endoscopic work-up of early Barrett's neoplasia. Endoscopy 2008;40:1000–7.
61. van Westreenen HL, Westerterp M, Sloof GW, et al. Limited additional value of positron emission tomography in staging oesophageal cancer. Br J Surg 2007; 94:1515–20.
62. Keswani RN, Early DS, Edmundowicz SA, et al. Routine positron emission tomography does not alter nodal staging in patients undergoing EUS-guided FNA for esophageal cancer. Gastrointest Endosc 2009;69:1210–7.

Photodynamic Therapy

Marta L. Davila, MD

KEYWORDS

- Photodynamic therapy • Barrett's esophagus
- Porfimer sodium • 5-aminolevulinic acid
- Esophageal adenocarcinoma

Photodynamic therapy (PDT) is one of the most widely studied ablative therapies used in the treatment of Barrett's esophagus (BE). BE is a condition in which the squamous epithelium of the esophagus is replaced by columnar, intestinal-type epithelium with goblet cells.[1] This metaplastic change often occurs as a consequence of chronic acid exposure. BE can progress to low-grade dysplasia (LGD), to high-grade dysplasia (HGD), and finally to adenocarcinoma.[1–4] BE is the primary risk factor for developing esophageal adenocarcinoma, with an estimated annual incidence of approximately 0.5%.[5] The highest risk for development of cancer is among patients with HGD. Approximately 30% to 35% of those patients progress to invasive cancer within 5 years.[6] Since 1975, there has been a dramatic increase in the incidence of esophageal adenocarcinoma in the United States, with adenocarcinoma being now more common than squamous cell carcinoma of the esophagus.[7]

The appropriate management of patients in whom HGD or early esophageal adenocarcinoma has been detected continues to be controversial. Historically, the standard of care for those patients was distal esophagectomy. However, esophagectomy is associated with significant morbidity and a 3% to 5% mortality rate, even when performed in high-volume expert centers.[8] Because of this, endoscopic ablative therapies have become attractive alternatives for these patients. Of the many endoscopic techniques capable of ablating columnar epithelium containing HGD, PDT is one of the most widely studied with some of the longest follow-up data.[9]

TECHNIQUE

PDT is a photochemical process that requires multiple steps to achieve tissue destruction. First, a photosensitizer drug is required. The only photosensitizer approved in the United States by the Food and Drug Administration for use in Barrett's HGD is porfimer sodium (Ps) (Photofrin, Wyeth-Ayerst Lederle Parenterals, Carolina,

The author has nothing to disclose.
Department of Gastroenterology, Hepatology and Nutrition, The University of Texas MD Anderson Cancer Center, 1515 Holcombe Boulevard, Unit 1466, Houston, TX 77030–4009, USA
E-mail address: mdavila@mdanderson.org

Gastrointest Endoscopy Clin N Am 21 (2011) 67–79
doi:10.1016/j.giec.2010.09.002
giendo.theclinics.com

PR, for Axcan ScandiPharm Inc). Ps is administered intravenously over 3 to 5 minutes at a dose of 2 mg/kg body weight. After systemic injection, the photosensitizer is absorbed by most tissues and retained at higher concentrations in neoplastic tissues.[10] Residual photosensitizer may remain in the skin for up to 4 to 8 weeks after injection, rendering the patient sensitive to ambient light and even strong indoor lighting for that period of time. The second step in the process is the application of light of proper power and wavelength to the target tissue. A variety of tunable dye lasers have been approved to activate photosensitizers. These laser units can generate the desired light and about 2 to 2.5 W of energy output. Visible red light at approximately 630 nm is typically used to activate the photosensitizer. The activated drug interacts with molecular oxygen leading to the generation of singlet oxygen. Subsequent radical reactions can form superoxide and hydroxyl radicals leading to cell membrane damage and apoptosis. It is important to note that laser treatment induces a photochemical, not a thermal effect. For endoscopic applications, illumination with laser light occurs 40 to 50 hours after injection with Ps.[11] The light is transmitted by optical fiber advanced through the accessory channel of an endoscope. The fibers come in several lengths to better match the length of the lesion being treated. Balloon diffusing fibers have also been used to deliver energy, but their use has not resulted in greater efficacy or in reduction of stricture formation.[12] For treatment of BE with HGD, the light dose recommended is 130 to 200 J/cm fiber. A second endoscopy is advised 96 to 120 hours after Ps injection to assess mucosal damage and degree of necrosis. If needed, a second light application can be administered to skipped or poorly treated areas.[11] The depth of injury of Ps at wavelength of 630 nm is approximately 5 to 6 mm, depending on tissue blood flow and oxygen levels (**Figs. 1** and **2**).[13]

There are other drugs, used mostly in Europe, for PDT applications, including 5-aminolevulinic acid (5-ALA) (Levulan, DUSA Pharmaceuticals, Wilmington, MA, USA), and m-tetrahydroxyphenyl chlorin (mTHPC) (Foscan, Biolitech, Pharma Ltd, Dublin, Ireland). ALA is present in virtually all human cells and is the first intermediate of the biochemical pathway resulting in heme synthesis. ALA differs from other drugs in that it is not a preformed photosensitizer but rather a precursor of the endogenously

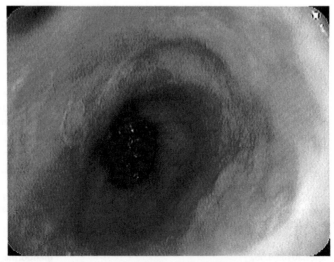

Fig. 1. Endoscopic view of Barrett's esophagus before photodynamic therapy.

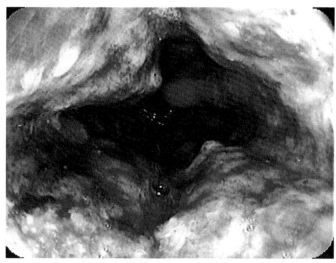

Fig. 2. Barrett's esophagus 48 hours after photodynamic therapy with porfimer sodium.

formed photosensitizer protoporphyrin IX.[14] Advantages of 5-ALA over Ps are the ability to administer it orally; the shorter duration of skin photosensitivity (24–48 hours); and the selective destruction of the mucosa that does not induce development of strictures.[15] 5-ALA is given at a dose of 30 to 60 mg/kg body weight orally in mineral water, orange juice, or lemonade, followed by light administration at 630 to 635 nm 4 to 6 hours later.[14,15] In 2007, 5-ALA was granted orphan drug status by the Food and Drug Administration for the treatment of patients with Barrett's HGD.

mTHPC has been used mostly for the treatment of advanced head and neck cancers and its use for BE-HGD or BE-adenocarcinoma is very limited. It is administered as a slow intravenous injection at a dose of 0.15 mg/kg. Patients are treated with red light (650–660 nm) or green light (511–514 nm) approximately 3 to 4 days after injection.[16,17] Skin photosensitivity may last for 2 to 3 weeks and there is a risk of stricture formation.[17]

PDT with Ps

Ps first received approval in the Unites States in 1995 for palliation of patients with advanced esophageal carcinoma. This approval was on the basis of a multicenter randomized controlled trial comparing PDT with neodymium:yttrium-aluminum-garnet (Nd:YAG) laser therapy. The study involved 218 patients and it showed both treatments were equally effective in improving dysphagia, but there were fewer complications in the group treated with PDT.[18] It was evident from the initial studies of esophageal cancer that treatment with PDT resulted in eradication of the segment of BE. This finding led to a number of studies using Ps-PDT for treatment of dysplastic Barrett's mucosa. Overholt and colleagues[19] reported their experience treating 100 patients with Ps-PDT, including 73 patients with BE-HGD, 14 patients with BE-LGD, and 13 patients with T1 to T2 adenocarcinoma. Patients were maintained on omeprazole and followed for a mean of 19 months. Small residual areas of Barrett's mucosa were treated with Nd:YAG laser. Seventy-three patients received one PDT treatment, twenty-two received two treatments, and five patients received three treatments. The authors found that 77% of cancers, 88% of BE-HGD, and 92% of BE-LGD were eradicated by PDT and focal thermal ablation. In 43% of patients, there was complete elimination of all Barrett's mucosa. The most common complication reported was stricture development in 34% of patients.[19]

Wolfsen and colleagues[20] retrospectively reviewed their experience with 48 patients (34 patients with BE-HGD and 14 patients with T1 cancers). All patients underwent only one course of Ps-PDT, and any residual Barrett's tissue was subsequently treated with argon plasma coagulator (APC). Complete, successful ablation of all BE-HGD and cancer was documented in 47 of 48 patients. One patient with persistent cancer underwent curative esophagectomy. Most frequent complications included strictures in 11 patients (23%); photosensitivity in 7 patients (15%); and esophageal perforation in 1 patient (2%), which resolved with supportive care.

Multiple other studies confirmed the benefits of Ps-PDT[21,22] and this led to the first randomized controlled treatment trial in BE with HGD.[11] The study included 30 sites and used a centralized expert pathology laboratory. A total of 208 patients were entered into the study and randomized in a 2:1 ratio to omeprazole plus Ps-PDT (138 patients) versus omeprazole alone (70 patients). Patients could receive up to three courses of PDT. Balloon diffusing fibers were used for the study, at a lower light dose of 130 J/cm. Follow-up consisted of endoscopy and four-quadrant biopsies every 2 cm performed every 3 months until four consecutive quarterly biopsies were negative for HGD, then every 6 months thereafter. The mean follow-up was 24 months. The primary outcome measure was complete ablation of HGD being noted at any time during the study period. Complete ablation of HGD was achieved in 77% (106 of 138) of patients in the omeprazole plus Ps-PDT group compared with 39% (27 of 70) in the omeprazole alone group ($P < .0001$). Complete eradication of all BE and dysplasia was seen in 52% of patients in the Ps-PDT group compared with 7% in the omeprazole group ($P < .0001$). There was also a significant difference in progression to cancer, with 13% of patients (N = 18) in the Ps-PDT group developing cancer compared with 28% (N = 20) in the omeprazole group. The most common Ps-PDT–related events were photosensitivity reactions (69%), esophageal strictures (36%), vomiting (32%), noncardiac chest pain (20%), pyrexia (20%), and dysphagia (19%). The authors concluded that Ps-PDT was an effective therapy for ablating BE-HGD and reducing the incidence of esophageal adenocarcinoma. The results of this study led the Food and Drug Administration to approve the use of Ps-PDT for the treatment of BE-HGD.

A 5-year follow-up of the original study[23] demonstrated the persistent superiority of Ps-PDT in eliminating HGD long-term (77% in the treatment group vs 39% in the omeprazole group). However, of the 102 patients eligible for long-term follow-up, only 61 patients (48 in the omeprazole plus Ps-PDT group and 13 in the omeprazole group) were enrolled in the long-term follow-up phase. The secondary outcome of progression to cancer remained significantly lower in the Ps-PDT group (15%) compared with 29% in the omeprazole group ($P = .027$). There was also a significantly longer time to progression to cancer favoring Ps-PDT ($P = .004$).

PDT has also been combined with endoscopic mucosal resection (EMR) for treatment of dysplasia and intramucosal cancers in BE. Seventeen patients with either T0 or T1 esophageal adenocarcinoma by EMR staging underwent PDT with Ps. At a median follow-up of 13 months, 16 patients (94%) remained in clinical and histologic remission. Three patients with positive mucosal resection margins remained cancer-free after PDT. Barrett's epithelium was eradicated in nine (53%) patients. Complications included self-limited bleeding after EMR in one patient (6%), and strictures after PDT in five patients (30%).[24] In a retrospective study of 24 patients who underwent EMR followed by PDT for early esophageal adenocarcinoma, 83% of patients (20 of 24) remained free of cancer at a mean follow-up of 1 year.[25]

A retrospective cohort study from Mayo Clinic evaluated the overall and cancer-free survival of two groups of patients with T1a esophageal adenocarcinoma in BE: one group was treated endoscopically with either EMR or EMR followed by Ps-PDT. The second group was treated with esophagectomy.[26] There were 132 patients in the endoscopy-treated group (75 with EMR alone and 57 with EMR plus Ps-PDT), and 46 in the surgically treated group. Patients treated endoscopically were older and had more medical comorbidities than those treated surgically. Remission was initially successful in 91% of patients treated with EMR plus Ps-PDT and in 96% of patients treated with EMR alone. Overall survival at 5 years was comparable in the endoscopy treated group (83%) and the surgical group (95%). Sixteen patients (12%) in the endoscopy group had recurrent carcinoma detected during follow-up, and all except one was managed by EMR. The presence of residual dysplastic BE was a significant factor predicting recurrent carcinoma on univariate analysis. The authors concluded that endoscopic therapy was a reasonable alternative to esophagectomy in patients with mucosal esophageal adenocarcinoma in BE.

There have been a few long-term studies evaluating predictors of response to Ps-PDT and risk factors for recurrence of dysplasia postablation. In one retrospective study of 116 patients with BE-HGD, and intramucosal and T1 adenocarcinoma treated with Ps-PDT, pretreatment length of BE was inversely correlated with successful ablation of all Barrett's epithelium. The presence of intramucosal adenocarcinoma (IMA) or T1 cancer was not associated with higher likelihood of treatment failure.[27] In another study evaluating 261 patients who underwent Ps-PDT with and without EMR, significant predictors of recurrence of dysplasia or neoplasia on multivariate analysis were older age, presence of residual nondysplastic BE, and history of smoking.[28] Biomarkers have also been examined as potential predictors of response to PDT. Using fluorescence in situ hybridization, one group found that p16 allelic loss predicted decreased response to PDT.[29]

A number of complications have been described with PDT (**Table 1**). Chest pain, nausea, dysphagia, and odynophagia are commonly reported within hours after laser light application. These are commonly treated with analgesics, both topical and systemic. These symptoms usually resolve within 1 to 2 weeks after therapy. Dehydration from poor oral intake needs to be closely monitored and treated, particularly in the elderly.[30]

Photosensitivity has been reported in as many as 69% of patients.[11] Because of the half-life of Ps and its absorption in cutaneous tissues, phototoxicity may last anywhere from 4 to 8 weeks. Patients are sensitive not only to sunlight but also to strong indoor lighting. Symptoms may range from mild erythema to blistering and bullae formation. Patients need to be advised on strict light-protective measures when outdoors, including use of clothing to cover all skin, hands, nose, ears, face, and scalp. By far, the most significant long-term complication of PDT is stricture

---

Table 1
Common complications reported with Porfimer sodium PDT

1. Cutaneous photosensitivity
2. Esophageal strictures
3. Chest pain
4. Dysphagia/Odynophagia
5. Nausea
6. Fever
7. Cardiac arrythmias
8. Pleural effusions

formation, reported in about one third of patients.[11,19] The reason strictures form after PDT with Ps is not known. It is possible that the deep tissue injury achieved by Ps-PDT leads to an aggressive fibrotic response that produces stricturing. Risk factors for development of strictures include history of previous esophageal stricture, performance of EMR before PDT, and more than one PDT application in one treatment session.[12] Another study identified the following independent predictors of stricture development: longer segment Barrett's, multiple PDT treatments, and evidence of intramucosal carcinoma before PDT.[31] The incidence of stricture formation can be decreased by using lower light doses ($\leq$115 J/cm), but this is at the expense of higher frequency of residual dysplasia or cancer in the treated area.[32] The use of centering balloons for laser light delivery[31] or oral steroids does not seem to reduce stricture formation.[33] Other less common complications include fever; vomiting; development of cardiac arrhythmias (particularly atrial fibrillation); and development of asymptomatic pleural effusions.[30]

One concern after PDT is the presence of buried intestinal metaplasia or malignancy underneath neosquamous epithelium.[19–22] In a study of 33 patients with BE-HGD or intramucosal carcinoma who underwent treatment with Ps-PDT, total buried BE was observed in 9 patients (27.3%) in pre-PDT biopsies and in 17 patients (51.5%) in post-PDT biopsies.[34] Buried dysplastic BE or carcinoma was observed in four patients in pre-PDT biopsies (12.1%) and in nine patients (27.3%) in post-PDT biopsies. In another study[35] involving 52 patients, not a single case of buried nondysplastic BE was noted pre-PDT. After PDT, buried nondysplastic BE was diagnosed in 12 biopsy levels (3.6% of 338 levels) of nine patients (17.3%). There was one patient (2%) with completely buried BE-HGD pre-PDT. After PDT, buried HGD-carcinoma was noted in 19 levels from 13 patients (25%). The occurrence of buried HGD-carcinoma after PDT was neither associated with the length of BE, the diffuseness of neoplasms, nor the presence of buried lesions before treatment.[35] In the largest study of squamous overgrowth and buried glands after Ps-PDT, Bronner and colleagues[36] analyzed the histologic specimens of 33,658 biopsies from the only randomized multicenter study of Ps-PDT for BE-HGD.[23] A total of 208 patients were randomly assigned (in a 2:1 ratio) to omeprazole plus Ps-PDT versus omeprazole alone. Patients underwent rigorous follow-up with four-quadrant jumbo esophageal biopsies every 2 cm throughout the pretreatment length of BE until four consecutive quarterly results were negative for HGD and then biannually up to 5 years or treatment failure. At baseline, squamous overgrowth was identified in 8 (5.8%) of 138 patients in the Ps-PDT group and 2 (2.9%) of 70 in the omeprazole group. After treatment, the percentage of biopsies with squamous overgrowth increased, but there was no significant difference between the Ps-PDT group (39 [30%] of 132) and the omeprazole group (22 [33%] of 67). On a per biopsy basis, squamous overgrowth was present in 114 (0.5%) of biopsies in the Ps-PDT group, and in 130 (1.3%) of biopsies in the omeprazole group, and this difference was not significant. The most advanced diagnosis was never concealed solely beneath squamous overgrowth (not even in a single patient), but it was always present in a surface biopsy taken according to protocol. The authors concluded that subsquamous overgrowth increased equally in the treatment group (omeprazole plus Ps-PDT) and control (omeprazole), and that previous studies using pretreatment biopsies as controls were inadequate in their design. When intensive biopsy surveillance is instituted, squamous overgrowth does not obscure the most advanced diagnosis. Treatment with Ps-PDT does not seem to present a long-term risk of failure to detect subsquamous dysplasia or carcinoma.[36]

PDT with 5-ALA

The first study of ALA-PDT for BE-HGD treated five patients with a median length of Barrett's segment of 5 cm.[37] Patients were given 60 mg/kg 5-ALA, followed 4 hours later by 630 nm of laser light at a dose of 90 to 150 J/cm². HGD was eradicated in all patients at 26 to 44 months of follow-up. In two patients, nondysplastic BE was noted underneath normal squamous mucosa. Gossner and colleagues[38] treated 32 patients (10 patients with BE-HGD and 22 patients with uT1N0M0 adenocarcinoma) with ALA-PDT at a dose of 60 mg/kg. Light was delivered at a wavelength of 635 nm with an energy dose of 150 J/cm². All patients were on 20 to 40 mg of omeprazole daily. HGD was eradicated in all patients (10 of 10) and mucosal cancer was eliminated in 17 (77%) of 22 patients at a mean follow-up of 9.9 months. All tumors less than or equal to 2 mm in thickness were completely ablated (17 of 17). Fifteen patients experienced nausea up to 6 hours after treatment. Mild increase in transaminase levels was documented in 21 of 32 patients; these values reached normal levels within a week.[38]

In the only double-blind, randomized, placebo-controlled study reported of ALA-PDT, 36 patients with BE and LGD were randomized to receive oral ALA (30 mg/kg) or placebo.[39] All patients were treated with green light (514 nm) at an energy density of 60 J/cm². Up to 6 cm of Barrett's were treated according to protocol. All patients were maintained on omeprazole, 20 mg daily. A response was seen in 16 (89%) of 18 patients in the ALA-PDT group, with a median decrease in area in the treated region of 30% (range, 0%–60%). In the placebo group, a median area decrease of 0% was seen (range, 0%–10%). This difference was statistically significant. Furthermore, there was complete eradication of LGD in all 18 patients in the ALA-PDT group, compared with only 6 (33%) of 18 in the placebo group ($P < .001$). The effects of treatment were maintained for up to 24 months.

The first long-term study of ALA-PDT in BE-HGD and T1a adenocarcinoma was reported by Pech and colleagues.[15] A total of 66 patients (35 with BE-HGD and 31 with intramucosal cancer) were treated with ALA-PDT at a dose of 60 mg/kg. Light was delivered at a wavelength of 635 nm with an energy dose of 150 J/cm². Median follow-up was 37 months. Complete remission was achieved in 34 (97%) of 35 patients with BE-HGD. Six patients (6 [18%] of 34) developed a recurrence or a metachronous lesion, but five of these underwent successful repeat treatment. In the IMA group, complete remission was achieved in all patients (31 of 31), but nine patients had recurrence of metachronous carcinoma (9 [29%] of 31). One patient was found to have HGD. Seven patients were successfully treated with ALA-PDT, and one went to surgery. One patient was not a surgical candidate and received palliative treatment 2 years later. Seven patients died during follow-up but no deaths were tumor related. The calculated 5-year survival was 97% in the BE-HGD group and 80% in the carcinoma group.[15]

Other studies of ALA-PDT have shown somewhat disappointing results. In a study from the Netherlands,[40] the authors set out to evaluate the efficacy of ALA-PDT in the eradication of residual neoplasia after previous EMR, and to assess the recurrence rate of neoplasia during follow-up. Patients were separated into two groups. Group A (11 patients) consisted of patients with proved residual HGD or early carcinoma after EMR. Group B (nine patients) consisted of patients with possible residual HGD or early carcinoma after EMR (no HGD or cancer other than in the resected focal lesion). Patients were given 5-ALA at a dose of 40 mg/kg. Ninety minutes to 4 hours after ingestion, red light was delivered at a wavelength of 630 nm for a total light dosage of 100 J/cm². The overall success rate was 15 (75%) of 20. There was a significant difference in success rate between group A (55%) and group B (100%) ($P = .03$). All patients had residual BE after PDT. The median regression percentage was 50%. Recurrence of HGD-carcinoma occurred in four patients (two in each group) after a median follow-up of 30 months. It is not clear as to what accounted for the low success rates reported in this study. A lower dose of oral 5-ALA (40 mg/kg) was used, compared with other studies that used 60 mg/kg.[15,37,38] There was a shorter interval between 5-ALA administration and light delivery (90–240 minutes as opposed to 240–360 minutes used in other studies). Thirdly, the total light dose in the study (100 J/cm^2) was lower than others have used.[37,38] Still, the authors argued, and rightly so, that there is no consensus about the optimal setting for any of these parameters.

It is clear there is a wide range of results reported with ALA-PDT, and there is also a high-recurrence rate in patients with early cancer.[15] This variability in results could be caused by multiple factors including 5-ALA dose; light dose; and type of light used (green vs red). In a nonrandomized light dose escalation study, 24 patients with BE-HGD received oral ALA at 60 mg/kg activated by different light doses.[41] The light dose can be expressed as either joule per centimeter length of treated esophagus or joule per square centimeter of the surface of the balloon. Light was administered as 500 J/cm (low dose, equivalent to 100 J/cm^2); 750 J/cm (medium dose, equivalent to 150 J/cm^2); 1000 J/cm (high dose, equivalent to 200 J/cm^2); or two 1000 J/cm treatments given 1 month apart (highest light dose, equivalent to 400 J/cm^2). The study revealed the highest light dose was significantly better than low and medium light dose for the eradication of HGD in BE. Six (75%) out of eight patients treated with the highest light dose (400 J/cm^2) compared with one (50%) out of two with a single high light dose treatment (200 J/cm^2), two (22%) out of nine receiving medium light dose (150 J/cm^2), and zero (0%) out of five receiving low light dose (100 J/cm^2), had successful long-term eradication of HGD.

In another study, the same group studied the optimal conditions for successful abla-tion of BE-HGD with ALA-PDT.[42] Initially, 16 patients were given 5-ALA at 30 mg/kg and randomized to either red (635 nm) or green light (512 nm) at a light dose of 200 J/cm^2. An interim analysis of the study revealed that HGD had been successfully erad-icated in only four patients (25%). After discussion with the ethics committee, the trial was restarted using 5-ALA at a dose of 60 mg/kg. Eleven patients were recruited and randomized to receive red or green light. All patients in the red light group had successful eradication of HGD, as opposed to one (20%) of five in the green light group ($P = .01$). After another ethics review, the study was extended to treat a further 21 patients with the most effective regimen of 60 mg/kg of 5-ALA, activated by red light at a light dose of 200 J/cm^2. At 36 months' follow-up, the success rate for HGD eradication in the patients treated with the best regimen was 89%. One patient had mild skin photosensitivity and no patients developed esophageal strictures. Two patients had self-limiting gastrointestinal bleeds, one of which required a blood trans-fusion. Nausea and vomiting were reported in over half of the patients and all patients receiving the 60 mg/kg dose showed minor, self-limiting elevation in liver function tests.[42] The authors concluded that the optimal regimen to treat BE-HGD was a 5-ALA dose of 60 mg/kg, activated by red light at a light dose of 200 J/cm^2.

In general, 5-ALA has an acceptable safety profile. The most common side effects reported include nausea, vomiting, transient rise in liver enzymes, mild transient photosensitivity, and hypotension.[14]

PDT with mTHPC

There are a limited number of studies evaluating the effectiveness of mTHPC for the treatment of BE-HGD and early esophageal cancer. In a study by Etienne and colleagues,[16] 12 patients with BE-HGD or IMA were enrolled to receive mTHPC-PDT. Four of the twelve patients had failed other therapies (including EMR, EMR plus APC, and Nd:YAG laser therapy). mTHPC was injected intravenously (0.15 mg/kg) 4 days before PDT with green light at 514 nm. The energy density administered was 75 J/cm^2. There were four visible lesions (one HGD, one IMA, and two HGD-IMA). There were 10 nonvisible lesions (six HGD, one IMA, and three HGD-IMA). Twenty PDT sessions were required to eradicate all lesions (nine lesions required only one treatment). The efficacy was 100%, with complete disappearance of HGD and IMA in all patients and the replacement of BE by squamous mucosa in the treated area. The mean follow-up was 34 months. Three patients died during the follow-up period of unrelated reasons. The most common adverse events reported included chest pain, fever, hiccups, asymptomatic bilateral pleural effusion, skin photosensitivity, phlebitis, and esophageal strictures.

In a pilot study, mTHPC was administered to 19 patients (7 HGD and 12 with early esophageal cancer).[17] The mean length of follow-up was 24 months. Successful eradication was seen using red light (652 nm) by diffuser in four of six patients with cancer and three of four with HGD. Using red light (652 nm) and a bare-tipped fiber resulted in eradication of cancer in only one of six patients. One patient in this group developed a fatal aortoesophageal fistula 10 weeks after PDT treatment. Another patient developed a tracheoesophageal fistula, successfully treated with a covered esophageal stent. This particular patient had received treatment with Nd:YAG laser 3 weeks before PDT. Both patients may have had biopsies early after PDT that may have contributed to these complications. None of the three patients with HGD treated with green light delivered by diffuser device had long-term eradication. Two patients developed esophageal strictures.[17]

This limited experience demonstrates that although mTHPC-PDT is a promising ablative therapy, optimal light and drug dosimetry are unknown. Further studies are needed to determine the ideal parameters for treatment under an accepted safety profile.

COST-EFFECTIVENESS

There have been a number of decision analyses studies evaluating the cost-effectiveness of PDT. One study[43] evaluated four different strategies for treatment of BE-HGD: (1) esophagectomy, (2) endoscopic surveillance, (3) PDT followed by esophagectomy for residual HGD, and (4) PDT followed by endoscopic surveillance for residual HGD. PDT followed by surveillance for residual HGD was the most effective strategy, with a quality-adjusted life expectancy of 12.31 quality-adjusted life years, but it also resulted in the greatest lifetime cost for an incremental cost-effectiveness of $47,410 per quality-adjusted life year. Both PDT and surveillance were effective and cost-effective treatments strategies if operative mortality was high, if cancer prevalence in HGD was low, or if surgery caused a marked reduction in quality of life. Another study[44] analyzed four different strategies including (1) no prevention, (2) elective surgical esophagectomy, (3) endoscopic ablation with PDT, and (4) surveillance endoscopy. Endoscopic ablation with PDT was the most effective strategy, yielding 15.5 discounted quality-adjusted life years compared with 15 for endoscopic surveillance and 14.9 for esophagectomy. Although endoscopic surveillance was less expensive than ablation, it was associated with shorter survival. A more recent study[45] created separate analyses for patients with no dysplasia, LGD, and HGD. The strategies compared were (1) no endoscopic surveillance, (2) endoscopic surveillance with ablation for incident dysplasia, (3) immediate ablation followed by endoscopic surveillance in all patients or limited to patients in whom metaplasia persisted, and (4) esophagectomy. Ablation modalities modeled included radiofrequency (RFA), APC, multipolar electrocoagulation, and PDT. Results revealed that endoscopic ablation for patients with HGD could increase life expectancy by 3 quality-adjusted years at an incremental cost of less than $6000 compared with no intervention. Ablation was estimated to be more effective and less costly than surveillance or esophagectomy for patients with BE-HGD. The effectiveness of the different ablation techniques seemed to be similar, with variation only in costs (PDT being more expensive). Ablation might also be preferred in subjects with LGD or no dysplasia, but the cost effectiveness depends on the long-term effectiveness of ablation and whether surveillance endoscopy can be discontinued after successful ablation.

SUMMARY

PDT is an effective method to eradicate HGD and to significantly reduce the risk of progression to cancer. There are advantages of PDT over other treatment modalities including ease of use; the need for fewer endoscopic sessions; and when compared with surgery, reduced morbidity, mortality, and cost. However, in the era of newer endoscopic ablative methods, PDT faces a number of challenges, such as the well-described complications of prolonged photosensitivity, high rate of stricture formation, and the severe pain and discomfort caused by the photochemical reaction.

To remain a viable clinical option, PDT candidates should be carefully selected to obtain more uniform results and minimize side effects. Dosimetry is one factor that needs further study. Most studies have focused on light dose, but there are other factors, including tissue properties of light scattering and absorption that need further evaluation. In addition, tissue photosensitizer levels should be systematically evaluated using available fluorescence spectroscopy techniques.[46,47] One group has suggested an additional variable in treatment outcome: esophageal thickness, as measured by endoscopic untrasound.[47] In that study, the total esophageal thickness for patients who had an ideal PDT response was significantly less than in those who appeared undertreated and had residual disease. Interestingly, the one patient who developed a post-PDT stricture had the smallest esophageal wall thickness.[47]

Future advances in PDT include the development of newer photosensitizers with more favorable characteristics, such as shorter half-life and absorption of light at higher wavelengths, which may result in shorter photosensitivity periods.

Although there are a large number of studies showing the efficacy of PDT for the treatment of BE-HGD and early esophageal adenocarcinoma, a number of unanswered questions remain. The future of PDT depends on careful patient selection and improving treatment parameters to maximize treatment outcomes while reducing complications.

REFERENCES

1. Haggitt RC. Barrett's esophagus, dysplasia, and adenocarcinoma. Hum Pathol 1994;25:982–93.
2. Weston AP, Sharma P, Topalovski M, et al. Long-term follow-up of Barrett's high-grade dysplasia. Am J Gastroenterol 2000;95:1888–93.
3. Reid BJ, Levine DS, Longton G, et al. Prediction of progression to cancer in Barrett's esophagus: baseline histology and flow cytometry identify low- and high-risk patient subsets. Am J Gastroenterol 2000;95:1669–76.

4. Buttar NS, Wang KK, Sebo TJ, et al. Extent of high-grade dysplasia in Barrett's esophagus correlated with risk of adenocarcinoma. Gastroenterology 2001; 120:1630–9.
5. Shaheen NJ, Crosby NA, Bozymski EM, et al. Is there publication bias in the reporting of cancer risk in Barrett's esophagus? Gastroenterology 2000;119:587–9.
6. Rastogi A, Puli S, El-Serag HB, et al. Incidence of esophageal adenocarcinoma in patients with Barrett's esophagus with high-grade dysplasia: a meta-analysis. Gastrointest Endosc 2008;67:394–8.
7. Pohl H, Welch HG. The role of overdiagnosis and reclassification in the marked increase of esophageal adenocarcinoma incidence. J Natl Cancer Inst 2005; 97:142–6.
8. Swisher SG, Deford L, Merriman KW, et al. Effect of operative volume on morbidity, mortality, and hospital use after esophagectomy for cancer. J Thorac Cardiovasc Surg 2000;119:1126–32.
9. Prasad GA, Wang KK, Buttar NS, et al. Long-term survival following endoscopic and surgical treatment of high-grade dysplasia in Barrett's esophagus. Gastroenterology 2007;132:1226–33.
10. Nishioka NS. Drug, light and oxygen: a dynamic combination in the clinic. Gastroenterology 1998;114:604–6.
11. Overholt BF, Lightdale CJ, Wang KK, et al. Photodynamic therapy with porfimer sodium for ablation of high-grade dysplasia in Barrett's esophagus: international, partially blinded, randomized phase III trial. Gastrointest Endosc 2005;62:488–98.
12. Prasad GA, Wang KK, Buttar NS, et al. Predictors of structure formation after photodynamic therapy for high-grade dysplasia in Barrett's esophagus. Gastrointest Endosc 2007;65:60–6.
13. Gross SA, Wolfsen HC. The role of photodynamic therapy in the esophagus. Gastrointest Endosc Clin N Am 2010;20:35–53.
14. Dunn J, Lovat L. Photodynamic therapy using 5-aminolaevulinic acid for the treatment of dysplasia in Barrett's oesophagus. Expert Opin Pharmacother 2008;9:851–8.
15. Pech O, Gossner L, May A, et al. Long-term results of photodynamic therapy with 5-aminolevulinic acid for superficial Barrett's cancer and high-grade intraepithelial neoplasia. Gastrointest Endosc 2005;62:24–30.
16. Etienne J, Dorme N, Bourg-Heckly G, et al. Photodynamic therapy with green light and m-tetrahydroxyphenyl chlorin for intramucosal adenocarcinoma and high-grade dysplasia in Barrett's esophagus. Gastrointest Endosc 2004;59:880–9.
17. Lovat LB, Jamieson NF, Novelli MR, et al. Photodynamic therapy with m-tetrahydroxyphenyl chlorin for high-grade dysplasia and early cancer in Barrett's columnar lined esophagus. Gastrointest Endosc 2005;62:617–23.
18. Lightdale CJ, Heier SK, Marcon NE, et al. Photodynamic therapy with porfimer sodium versus thermal ablation therapy with Nd:YAG laser for palliation of esophageal cancer: a multicenter randomized trial. Gastrointest Endosc 1995;42: 507–12.
19. Overholt BF, Panjehpour M, Haydek JM. Photodynamic therapy for Barrett's esophagus: follow-up in 100 patients. Gastrointest Endosc 1999;49:1–7.
20. Wolfsen HC, Woodward TA, Raimondo M. Photodynamic therapy for dysplastic Barrett's esophagus and early esophageal adenocarcinoma. Mayo Clin Proc 2002;77:1176–81.
21. Overholt BF, Panjehpour M, Halberg DL. Photodynamic therapy for Barrett's esophagus with dysplasia and/or early stage carcinoma: long term results. Gastrointest Endosc 2003;58:183–8.

22. Wolfsen HC, Hemminger LL, Wallace MB, et al. Clinical experience of patients undergoing photodynamic therapy for Barrett's dysplasia or cancer. Aliment Pharmacol Ther 2004;20:1125–31.
23. Overholt BF, Wang KK, Burdick S, et al. Five-year efficacy and safety of photodynamic therapy with Photofrin in Barrett's high-grade dysplasia. Gastrointest Endosc 2007;66:460–8.
24. Buttar NS, Wang KK, Lutzke LS, et al. Combined endoscopic mucosal resection and photodynamic therapy for esophageal neoplasia within Barrett's esophagus. Gastrointest Endosc 2001;54:682–8.
25. Pacifico RJ, Wang KK, Wongkeesong LM, et al. Combined endoscopic mucosal resection and photodynamic therapy versus esophagectomy for management of early adenocarcinoma in Barrett's esophagus. Clin Gastroenterol Hepatol 2003;1: 252–7.
26. Prasad GA, Wu TT, Wigle DA, et al. Endoscopic and surgical treatment of mucosal (T1a) esophageal adenocarcinoma in Barrett's esophagus. Gastroenterology 2009;137:815–23.
27. Yachimski P, Puricelli WP, Nishioka NS. Patient predictors of histopathologic response after photodynamic therapy of Barrett's esophagus with high-grade dysplasia or intramucosal carcinoma. Gastrointest Endosc 2009;69:205–12.
28. Badreddine RJ, Prasad GA, Wang KK, et al. Prevalence and predictors of recurrent neoplasia after ablation of Barrett's esophagus. Gastrointest Endosc 2010; 71:697–703.
29. Prasad GA, Wang KK, Halling KC, et al. Utility of biomarkers in prediction of response to ablative therapy in Barrett's esophagus. Gastroenterology 2008; 135:370–9.
30. Wang KK, Nijhawan PK. Complications of photodynamic therapy in gastrointestinal disease. Gastrointest Endosc Clin N Am 2000;10:487–95.
31. Yachimski P, Puricelli WP, Nishioka NS. Patient predictors of esophageal stricture development after photodynamic therapy. Clin Gastroenterol Hepatol 2008;6: 302–8.
32. Panjehpour M, Overholt BF, Phan MN, et al. Optimization of light dosimetry for photodynamic therapy of Barrett's esophagus: efficacy vs. incidence of stricture after treatment. Gastrointest Endosc 2005;61:13–8.
33. Panjehpour M, Overholt BF, Haydek JM, et al. Results of photodynamic therapy for ablation of dysplasia and early cancer in Barrett's esophagus and effect of oral steroids on stricture formation. Am J Gastroenterol 2000;95:2177–84.
34. Ban S, Mino M, Nishioka NS, et al. Histopathologic aspects of photodynamic therapy for dysplasia and early adenocarcinoma arising in Barrett's esophagus. Am J Surg Pathol 2004;28:1466–73.
35. Mino-Kenudson M, Ban S, Ohana M, et al. Buried dysplasia and early adenocarcinoma arising in Barrett esophagus after porfimer-photodynamic therapy. Am J Surg Pathol 2007;31:403–9.
36. Bronner MP, Overholt BF, Taylor SL, et al. Squamous overgrowth is not a safety concern for photodynamic therapy for Barrett's esophagus with high-grade dysplasia. Gastroenterology 2009;136:56–64.
37. Barr H, Sheperd NA, Dix A, et al. Eradication of high-grade dysplasia in columnar-lined (Barrett's) oesophagus by photodynamic therapy with endogenously generated protoporphyrin IX. Lancet 1996;348:584–5.
38. Gossner L, Stolte M, Sroka R, et al. Photodynamic ablation of high-grade dysplasia and early cancer in Barrett's esophagus by means of 5-aminolevulinic acid. Gastroenterology 1998;114:448–55.

39. Ackroyd R, Brown NJ, Davis MF, et al. Photodynamic therapy for dysplastic Barrett's oesophagus: a prospective, double blind, randomized, placebo controlled trial. Gut 2000;47:612–7.
40. Peters F, Kara M, Rosmolen W, et al. Poor results of 5-aminolevulinic acid-photo-dynamic therapy for residual high-grade dysplasia and early cancer in Barrett esophagus after endoscopic resection. Endoscopy 2005;37:418–24.
41. Mackenzie GD, Jamieson NF, Novelli MR, et al. How light dosimetry influences the efficacy of photodynamic therapy with 5-aminolaevulinic acid for ablation of high-grade dysplasia in Barrett's esophagus. Lasers Med Sci 2008;23:203–10.
42. Mackenzie GD, Dunn JM, Selvasekar CR, et al. Optimal conditions for successful ablation of high-grade dysplasia in Barrett's oesophagus using aminolaevulinic acid photodynamic therapy. Lasers Med Sci 2009;24:729–34.
43. Vij R, Triadafilopoulos G, Owens DK, et al. Cost-effectiveness of photodynamic therapy for high-grade dysplasia in Barrett's esophagus. Gastrointest Endosc 2004;60:739–56.
44. Shaheen NJ, Inadomi JM, Overholt BF, et al. What is the best management strategy for high-grade dysplasia in Barrett's oesophagus? A cost-effectiveness analysis. Gut 2004;53:1736–44.
45. Inadomi JM, Somsouk MA, Madanick RD, et al. A cost-utility analysis of ablative therapy for Barrett's esophagus. Gastroenterology 2009;136:2101–14.
46. Wang KK, Lutzke L, Borkenhagen L, et al. Photodynamic therapy for Barrett's esophagus: does light still have a role? Endoscopy 2008;40:1021–5.
47. Gill KR, Wolfsen HC, Preyer NW, et al. Pilot study on light dosimetry variables for photodynamic therapy of Barrett's esophagus with high-grade dysplasia. Clin Cancer Res 2009;15:1830–6.

Endoscopic Resection

Oliver Pech, MD, PhD*, Hendrik Manner, MD, PhD,
Christian Ell, MD, PhD

KEYWORDS

- Endoscopic resection • Barrett's esophagus
- High-grade intraepithelial neoplasia
- Endoscopic submucosal dissection

Endoscopic resection (ER) of early neoplastic lesions has become increasingly important in recent years, both as a diagnostic tool for the staging of esophageal carcinoma and as a method of performing definitive treatment when the cancer meets certain criteria in which the risk of lymph node metastasis is negligible.[1] For many years, surgery was considered to be the treatment of choice, even in patients with high-grade intraepithelial neoplasia (HGIN) or mucosal carcinoma, but it is associated with a 30-day mortality of 2% to 5% and with significant morbidity in 30% to 50% of cases, even in high-volume centers.[2–6]

Because of these alarming data, local treatment methods have been introduced and investigated in several studies on early Barrett's neoplasia. In contrast to ablative treatment methods, such as photodynamic therapy (PDT), argon plasma coagulation (APC), cryotherapy, and radiofrequency ablation (RFA), ER allows histologic assessment of the resected specimen to assess the depth of infiltration of the tumor (pT1m1–4; pT1sm1–3) and whether an infiltration of lymph (L-status) or blood vessels (V-status) is present. In addition, the pathologist can provide important information about the freedom from neoplasia at the lateral and (more importantly) basal margins, imitating the surgical situation.[1] These significant advantages of ER are the main reason why ER should be preferred over all ablative treatment methods whenever possible, especially keeping in mind the low accuracy of endoscopic ultrasound regarding local tumor staging.[7–11]

ER TECHNIQUES

"Endoscopic resection" is the general term for the different resection techniques used to treat neoplastic and uncertain lesions in the gastrointestinal tract. The aim of ER must always be complete resection of the mucosal and submucosal layer down to the lamina muscularis propria. The term "endoscopic mucosal resection" or "mucosectomy" is also widely used; however, it is misleading because significant

Department of Internal Medicine 2, HSK Wiesbaden, Ludwig-Erhard-Strasse 100, 65199,
Wiesbaden, Germany
* Corresponding author.
E-mail address: oliver.pech@t-online.de

Gastrointest Endoscopy Clin N Am 21 (2011) 81–94
doi:10.1016/j.giec.2010.10.001
1052-5157/11/$ – see front matter © 2011 Elsevier Inc. All rights reserved.

proportions of the submucosal layer are also resected, which is important in the case of submucosal infiltration of the tumor.

ER with a Ligation Device

A widely used method is ER with a ligation device, also used for ligation of esophageal varices. With this method, the target lesion is sucked into the cylinder of the ligation device and a rubber band is then released to create a pseudopolyp that has the rubber band at its base. Prior submucosal injection of saline is usually not necessary. After this, the endoscope is withdrawn to remove the ligation cylinder. Afterward, the endoscope is reintroduced and the pseudopolyp is resected with a reusable snare underneath the rubber band to achieve larger resection specimens.

Several ligation devices are available. In addition to single-use devices, available ligation devices include a reusable ligator, with which similar results can be achieved at reduced cost. Ligation devices with multiple rubber bands are also available to allow several ligations to be performed in a single session without having to withdraw the endoscope. Another useful development is a ligation cylinder that has six rubber bands and a facility for advancing a snare through the working channel of a regular endoscope. This enables the endoscopist to perform up to six resections without having to withdraw and reintroduce the endoscope. This device is widely used for piecemeal resections of larger neoplastic lesions.

ER with a Transparent Cap

The cap technique was introduced by Inoue and Endo[12] almost 20 years ago for resection of early neoplastic lesions. In ER with the cap technique, a specially developed transparent plastic cap is attached to the end of the endoscope. After submucosal injection under the target lesion, usually with a saline–epinephrine solution, the lesion is sucked into the cap and resected with a diathermy snare that has previously been loaded onto a specially designed groove on the lower edge of the cap. Preloading of the snare can be done in the gastric antrum by applying slight suction to the mucosa and carefully advancing the snare until it is placed exactly in the rim at the distal margin of the cap. Prior marking of the borders of the lesion either with electrocautery using the tip of the snare or an APC probe is recommended, because injecting underneath a discrete neoplastic lesion often makes it difficult to identify the borders of the target lesion afterward.

ER with a ligation device and ER with the cap can be performed in the esophagus with similar results and complication rates. A prospective randomized trial with 100 consecutive ERs in 70 patients comparing ER with a reusable ligation device with ER with the cap was able to demonstrate that there is no difference regarding size of the resection specimens, the resection area, and complication rate.[13] One minor bleeding incident occurred in each group, but no severe complications were seen. However, another retrospective study from the Amsterdam group showed that ER with a multiband ligator was faster and safer than cap resection. Mild bleeding occurred significantly more often after cap ER (20% vs 6%).[14]

The major drawback of ER with the suck-and-cut technique seems to be that only small lesions with a diameter of less than 20 mm can be resected en bloc with tumor-free lateral margins. Ulcerated lesions often have fibrosis attaching the submucosa to the lamina muscularis propria, often resulting in failure of the lesion to lift. In these cases, ER is not advisable, or should only be performed with caution. Larger lesions can usually be resected completely with the piecemeal technique, but this method seems to be associated with a higher recurrence rate probably because of small neoplastic residues resulting from insufficient overlapping of the resection areas. For piecemeal ER the ligation device or cap has to be placed at the margin of the prior resection area and careful suction has to be applied (**Fig. 1**). The endoscopist has to be very careful to avoid small neoplastic remnants between the resection areas. On the other side, there is a danger of sucking the proper muscle layer of the previous resection into the pseudopolyp leading to a perforation. To minimize the risk of complications and of insufficient resection, only experienced endoscopists in high-volume centers should perform this procedure. En bloc resection allows more accurate histologic evaluation of the neoplastic lesion, especially of the lateral and basal margins. A new resection technique, endoscopic submucosal dissection (ESD), was therefore developed.

ESD

The ESD procedure in the treatment of early gastric cancer was first described by Hosokawa and Yoshida[15] and Ono and colleagues[16] with a method using an insulated-tip knife to obtain a large resection specimen with the neoplasm resected en bloc (**Fig. 2**). Once the borders of a neoplastic lesion have been adequately visualized the borders are marked with electrocautery at a distance of 5 to 10 mm from the margin of the carcinoma. After this, submucosal injection of fluid is performed to elevate the lesion from the muscular layer, and the mucosa surrounding the lesion is circumferentially cut outside the markings. Finally, the submucosal connective tissue is dissected with a dedicated knife. Visible vessels can be coagulated to prevent bleeding. The fluid used for submucosal injection can be isotonic saline solution, a solution of hyaluronic acid with or without glycerol, or 20% glucose or hypertonic saline with epinephrine.[1] Some endoscopists add a dye, such as indigo

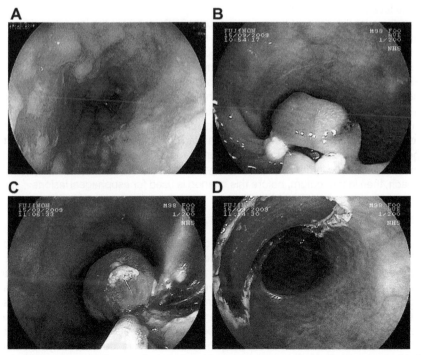

Fig. 1. Radical endoscopic resection of a large Barrett's cancer with the ligation device (A–D).

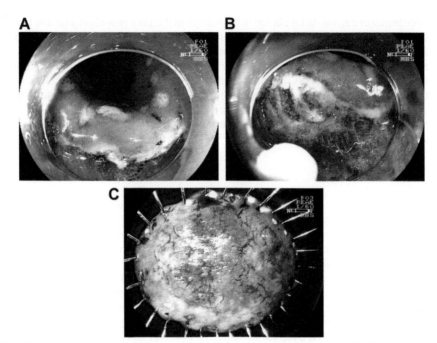

Fig. 2. Endoscopic submucosal dissection of a mucosal Barrett's cancer (A–C).

carmine, to the solution to facilitate discrimination of the submucosal from the proper muscle layer.

A wide variety of different knives are used for ESD, including the insulated-tip knife, hook knife, flex knife, needle-knife, triangle-tip knife, flush knife, and hybrid knife. With the flush and hybrid knife submucosal injection and dissection can be performed at the same time without changing the instruments.

ESD is not only used for gastric cancers but also for esophageal, colorectal, and duodenal neoplastic lesions. The size of the resected specimen obtained with ESD can extend to more than 10 cm in diameter, but this fascinating new method is associated with a substantial complication rate, including perforations requiring surgery, long procedure times of up to several hours, a slow learning curve, and a high degree of operator dependency. The endoscopist should first start to practice ESD in models to become familiar with this technique. Afterward, they should start with ESD procedures in the stomach, then in the rectum, before this method is used for esophageal lesions.

INDICATIONS AND RESULTS OF ER IN HGIN AND EARLY BARRETT'S CANCER

ER is the treatment of choice in high-grade dysplasia (HGD) and early mucosal cancer in Barrett's esophagus because the risk for lymph node and distant metastasis is almost absent. Large series from several groups demonstrate the safety and efficacy of this treatment approach even after long-term follow-up.[17–23] Risk stratification should be performed in accordance with known risk factors, such as grade of differentiation, lymph vessel or venous infiltration, and the infiltration depth of the carcinoma (m1–m3/m4). From the authors' center's experience with 899 patients with mucosal Barrett's cancer treated endoscopically only 0.34% have developed lymph node metastasis. Those patients usually had lymph vessel invasion on histology (L1 status).

Thirty-eight patients with mucosal Barrett's cancer have been referred to the surgical unit for esophageal resection because of unfavorable conditions for ER or high-risk situation after diagnostic ER. Among those negatively selected patients three (7.8%) were found to have metastatic nodes. The overall risk for lymph node metastasis in mucosal Barrett's cancer in the authors' center was 0.6%. However, a strong predictor for lymphatic spread was lymph vessel infiltration. Therefore, all patients should be referred for esophageal resection in case of a L1 situation.

Submucosal invasion goes along with a significantly increased lymph node risk of up to 41% and it strongly correlates with the infiltration depth. Cancer invading the upper third of the submucosa (pT1sm1) has a risk varying between 0% and 21%. Cancer invading the mid and lower submucosa (pT1sm2/3) goes along with metastatic lymph nodes in 36% to 54%.[2,24–27] These data are mainly from older retrospective surgical series in a time when exact determination of the tumor infiltration depth had little clinical relevance. In contrast to ER specimen that are sliced every 1 to 2 mm, surgical resection specimens were routinely cut in 5-mm slices. This explains that deeper infiltrating parts of the tumor might have been missed, underestimating invasion depth. Reported rates of lymph node metastasis might have corresponded with deeper invading cancers. Further important risk factors, such as differentiation grade and lymphatic and vascular invasion, were usually not reported making it impossible to draw final conclusions from these series. Some data are suggesting that ER can safely be performed in so-called "low-risk" submucosal cancer (sm1-cancer, G1/2, L0, V0) but larger series are awaited to generally recommend ER in these patients.[2,26]

Clinical Outcome of ER

The relevant publications on ER of early Barrett's neoplasia are summarized in **Table 1**. The first report on ER in 64 patients with early carcinoma or HGIN arising in Barrett's esophagus was published in 2000.[17] Complete remission was achieved with ER in 82.5% of cases (97% in the low-risk group and 59% in the high-risk group) in the study. During a mean follow-up period of 12 months, recurrences or metachronous lesions were observed in 14% of patients, who underwent successful endoscopic retreatment.

In a further study 115 patients with HGIN (N = 19) and early Barrett's carcinoma (N = 96) were treated with ER (N = 70); PDT (N = 32); a combination of the two (N = 10); or APC (N = 3).[28] Complete remission could be achieved in 98% of the patients, but metachronous neoplasia was found in 31% during a mean follow-up period of 34 months.

Until 2006, no long-term results for ER in patients with early Barrett's neoplasia were available. Ell and colleagues[18] provided excellent long-term results for ER in 100 consecutive patients with low-risk mucosal Barrett's cancer. Complete remission was achieved in 99% of cases, and the 5-year overall survival rate was 98%. None of the patients died of Barrett's neoplasia in the study, and minor bleeding occurred in 11 cases. Metachronous lesions were observed in only 11% after 36.7 months. This study of ER in a highly selected cohort of patients with low-risk Barrett's carcinoma does not reflect the general population of patients with Barrett's neoplasia, but clearly underlines the safety and efficacy of the method in a highly specialized center.

The authors' group recently published the largest series on endoscopic treatment of early Barrett's neoplasia in 349 patients.[19] A total of 61 had HGIN and 288 presented with mucosal carcinoma. ER was performed in 279 patients, PDT with 5-aminolevulinic acid as a photosensitizer in 55 patients, and both methods were combined in 13 patients for treatment of neoplastic Barrett's esophagus. Treatment was highly

Table 1
Endoscopic resection in early Barrett's neoplasia

Author (year)	Patient Number	ER Technique	Complications	% Complete Response	Follow-up (months)	% Recurrence/ Metachronous NPL
Ell et al[17] (2000)	64 (3 HGIN, 61 T1m)	ER-L	Minor bleeding 12.5%	82.5	12	14
Nijhawan & Wang[42] (2000)	17 (4 HGIN, 13 T1m)	L&C, ER-L (7 PDT, 2 OP)	0%	100	14.6	0
Buttar et al[43] (2001)	17 (7 BE/LGIN/HGIN, 10 T1m/T1sm)	ER-L + PDT	Minor bleeding 6% Strictures 30%	94	13	0
May et al[28] (2002)	115 (19 HGIN, 95 T1m, 11 T1sm)	66 ER-L, 32 PDT, 9 ER + PDT, 3 APC	Minor bleeding 7.5% Strictures 4.5%	98	31	30
Behrens et al[44] (2005)	44 HGIN	14 ER-L 27 PDT	Minor bleeding 9.3%	97.7	38	17.1
Conio et al[45] (2005)	39 (5 LGIN, 27 HGIN, 2 T1m, 5 T1sm)	ER-C	Bleeding 10.3%	94	34.9	3
Peters et al[33] (2008)	33 (3 BE, 8 HGIN, 15 T1m, 7 T1sm)	ER-C	Minor bleeding 45%	79	19	19
Ell et al[18] (2007)	100 T1m	ER-L	Minor bleeding 10%	98	36.7	11
Pech et al[19] (2008)	349 (61 HGIN, 288 T1m)	279 ER-L, 55 PDT, 13 ER + PDT, 2 APC	Major bleeding 0.6% Minor bleeding 11.5% Strictures 4.3%	96.6	63	21.5
Manner et al[26] (2008)	21 T1sm1	ER-L	Minor bleeding	95	62	29
Thomas et al[46] (2009)	16 (13 HGIN, 3 T1m)	ER-L	Bleeding 18.7%	87.5	8	0
Pech et al[47] (2009)	1059 (106 HGIN, 819 T1m, 134 T1sm)	917 ER-L 81 PDT, 33 ER + PDT, 28 APC	10 minor bleeding Strictures 6%	95	56	13.5

Abbreviations: BE, Barrett's esophagus; ER-C, ER with the cap technique; ER-L, ER with a ligation device; L&C, lift & cut; LGIN, low-grade intraepithelial neoplasia; NPL, neoplasia; OP, surgery.

effective with a remission rate of 96.6%. During a follow-up of more than 5 years, however, metachronous and recurrent neoplasia was observed in 21.5% of cases. Most patients were retreated successfully and long-term complete response was achieved in 94.5%. Long-term survival of patients treated for Barrett's neoplasia in this series did not significantly differ from that of the normal German population with the same age and gender distribution.

Those results clearly demonstrated that ER is safe and effective in HGD and mucosal Barrett's cancer even after a 5-year follow-up, but recurrences or metachronous neoplasia have been shown to be the major problem with endoscopic therapy in early Barrett's neoplasia. However, successful repeat endoscopic treatment is usually possible in almost all patients. The reasons for the high rate of recurrence seem to be a percentage of undetected neoplasia in the residual Barrett's segment after treatment and, more importantly, the fact that the residual Barrett's metaplasia seems to have an increased risk of malignant transformation because of genetic abnormalities not influenced by focal endoscopic treatment. Risk factors for recurrence or metachronous neoplasia were as follows: long-segment Barrett's esophagus, piecemeal resection, a long treatment phase of more than 10 months, and multifocal neoplasia at baseline. However, the results were also able to demonstrate that ablative therapy of the remaining nondysplastic Barrett's epithelium after successful ER could significantly decrease the risk. Those results were confirmed in a prospective randomized trial by the authors' group comparing ER of all neoplastic lesions followed by ablation of the nondysplastic Barrett's epithelium with ER and follow-up.[29] The study had to be prematurely aborted after inclusion of 56 patients because recurrence rate was 0% in the APC arm and 29.6% in the follow-up arm ($P = .003$) after a mean follow-up of 19.5 months. The data clearly demonstrate that ablative treatment of the remaining nondysplastic Barrett's epithelium after successful ER of all detectable neoplastic lesions can significantly reduce the recurrence rate and should always be performed.

ER can also be combined with RFA as demonstrated by the Amsterdam group. Two recently published studies by Gondrie and colleagues[30,31] combined ER of visible neoplastic lesions with circumferential and focal RFA of the remaining Barrett's esophagus containing HGIN in 23 patients. Ablation without prior ER was performed in 10 patients with flat HGIN. Complete elimination of neoplasia and Barrett's metaplasia was possible in all of the 23 included patients and none of the 836 biopsies of the neosquamous mucosa contained subsquamous Barrett's esophagus.

RFA seems to be the ideal addendum to ER for ablation of the remaining nondysplastic Barrett's epithelium after successful resection of all localizable HGIN and adenocarcinoma. There is no study, however, comparing RFA with APC for this indication, making final conclusions difficult.

A removal of all neoplastic lesions by ER before ablation provides a specimen that can be evaluated by the pathologist regarding infiltration depth and risk factors for lymphatic spread. RFA or APC treatment of HGIN diagnosed on biopsy, even in flat mucosal, harbors the risk of undertreatment. Also, flat neoplastic lesions have a risk for submucosal infiltration, as demonstrated in two large series.[32,33] Especially, slightly depressed neoplasias have a 25% risk of being associated with submucosal infiltration.

Complete Circumferential ER

Another concept to reduce the rate of recurrent malignancy after successful ER is complete circumferential ER to eradicate the entire Barrett's mucosa at risk. Several studies investigated this concept (**Table 2**) .Seewald and colleagues[34] first described circumferential ER in 12 patients with early Barrett's neoplasia. The complete Barrett's

Table 2
Radical ER of Barrett's esophagus

Author (year)	Patient Number	ER Technique	Complications	% Complete Response	Follow-up (months)	% Recurrence/ Metachronous NPL
Seewald et al[34] (2003)	12 (3 BE/LGIN, 5 HGIN, 4 MC)	Circumferential L&C	Strictures 17% Minor bleeding 33%	100	9	0
Giovannini et al[35] (2004)	21 (12 HGIN, 9 MC)	Semicircumf. L&C	Bleeding 19%	86	18	11
Soehendra et al[36] (2006)	10 (2 HGIN, 8 T1m)	Circumferential ER-L	Minor bleeding 20% Strictures 70% (1 death after dilatation)	90	—	—
Peters et al[20] (2006)	39 (3 BE, 1 LGIN, 18 HGIN, 12 MC, 3 SMC)	Circumferential ER-C	0%	100	14.6	0
Larghi et al[37] (2007)	17 (7 BE/LGIN/HGIN, 10 T1m/T1sm)	ER-L + PDT	Minor bleeding 6% Strictures 30%	94	13	0
Lopes et al[38] (2007)	41 (18 HGIN, 23 T1m)		Bleeding 19.5% Perforation 5% Strictures 2.5%		31.6	12.5
Chennat et al[21] (2009)	49 (33 HGIN, 14 T1m, 2 T1sm)	ER-C, ER-L, L&C	Strictures 37%	65 (29 under treatment)	22.9	0
Pouw et al[22] (2010)	169 (12 BE, 10 LGIN, 71 HGIN, 69 T1m, 7 T1sm)	ER-C, ER-L, L&C	Bleeding 2.4% Perforation 2.4% Strictures 49.7%	97.5 (1 tumor-related death)	32	2.3

Abbreviations: BE, Barrett's esophagus; ER-C, ER with the cap technique; ER-L, ER with a ligation device; L&C, lift & cut; LGIN, low-grade intraepithelial neoplasia; MC, mucosal cancer; NPL, neopalsia; SMC, submucosal cancer.

segment was resected in one to five sessions, with a median of five ERs per session (range, 1–19). Complications occurred in six cases (four cases of bleeding and two strictures), all of which were managed endoscopically. The median follow-up in this small series was 9 months, and no recurrences were observed.

Another study by Giovannini and colleagues[35] also investigated the concept of complete circumferential ER of the entire Barrett's segment. Twelve patients with HGIN and nine with mucosal cancer were included in the study. ER was performed in two sessions. In the first session, the lesion and the surrounding half of the Barrett's segment was removed by ER. In a second session 1 month later, the other half of the segment was resected to prevent stricture formation, which was observed in none of the patients in the series. Complete remission of cancer was achieved in 18 cases (86%); the three remaining patients underwent surgery (N = 1) or chemoradiotherapy (N = 2). Complete removal of the Barrett's epithelium was only possible in 75% of cases, and malignancy recurred in two patients (11%) during a mean follow-up period of 18 months.

Similar results were achieved by the Amsterdam group.[20] Complete eradication of early neoplasia was achieved in all 37 patients treated in a median number of three sessions, and complete removal of all Barrett's mucosa was achieved in 33 patients (89%). Symptomatic stenoses occurred in 26% of patients; further complications observed were one perforation and one case of delayed bleeding, all managed endoscopically. No recurrences had been observed after 11 months.

The largest United States series on circumferential ER published by Chennat and colleagues[21] reported on the results in 33 patients with HGD and 16 patients with mucosal cancer. Complete eradication of neoplasia and Barrett's epithelium could be achieved in all except of 1 of the 32 patients who completed treatment. Symptomatic esophageal stenosis was developed by 37% of patients, but all could be managed endoscopically. No further severe complications were observed.

A European multicenter trial included 169 patients with early Barrett's neoplasia.[23] Stepwise radical ER was performed in four tertiary referral centers to eradicate Barrett's esophagus with neoplasia. Complete eradication of neoplasia and Barrett's epithelium could be achieved in 97.6% and 85.2% of patients, respectively. One patient showed progression of cancer and died from metastatic disease and four patients developed recurrence after a median follow-up of 32 months. Symptomatic esophageal stenosis was also a major problem in this series and was observed in almost 50% of patients.

One of the major advantages of radical ER of neoplastic Barrett's esophagus is the possibility that the whole Barrett's segment can be evaluated by the pathologist to detect and stage even neoplasia not visualized endoscopically. The downside of complete radical ER of the whole Barrett's segment is the high stricture rate associated with this method requiring repeated dilatation. Therefore, a combination of ER of all visible neoplastic lesions followed by thermal ablation of the remaining Barrett's epithelium seems to be the better treatment strategy combining the positive effect of tissue acquisition with a low complication rate associated with ablation.[19,22,29]

ESD

There is almost no experience with ESD in patients with early Barrett's neoplasia. In a smaller series published by Kakushima and colleagues,[39] ESD was performed in 30 patients with tumors of the esophagogastric junction. Only four of the patients had early Barrett's cancer. The average maximum diameters of the lesions and resected specimens were 22.4 and 40.6 mm, respectively. The R0 resection rate was 97% (29 of 30). Histology revealed lymph vessel invasion in five patients and submucosal invasion deeper than 500 μm also in five cases. Another series from Japan reported on ESD of superficial adenocarcinoma of the esophagogastric junction.[40] ESD was performed in 25 cancers in 24 patients. The en bloc resection rate was 100% in this series but only 72% of lesions were judged as a curative resection. No recurrences were observed in this group during a median follow-up of 30.1 months.

The results of a prospective randomized trial from Belgium comparing cap ER with ESD in patients with early Barrett's neoplasia is only published in abstract form.[41] Twenty-five patients were included in each group. Larger neoplastic lesions in the ER group had to be resected in piecemeal technique and therefore tumor free margins (R0) of the resected specimens were only observed in 24%. In contrast, R0 resection rate was 64% in the ESD group. However, complete resection of all neoplasias was achieved in both groups and recurrences were observed in both groups after a follow-up of 15 months. Perforations occurred in two patients in the ESD group and one patient in the ER group. Strictures were observed in significantly more patients in the ESD group than in the ER group (44% vs 20%).

Although ESD is theoretically the ideal treatment technique in patients with early Barrett's neoplasia, data so far do not support its use for Barrett's neoplasia outside prospective studies. The outcome after ESD does not seem to be better than after conventional ER and data from Western centers are scarce. It is questionable whether ESD, a demanding, time-consuming technique with a flat learning curve and a high complication rate can significantly improve the results of ER combined with ablation already achieved by many Western groups (remission rates 90%–100%).

Surgery Versus ER

There are only scarce data comparing radical esophageal resection with ER. The Mayo group has recently published a paper where they compared a cohort of patients with mucosal Barrett's cancer treated by ER with another cohort treated by esophageal resection.[6] The design was a retrospective cohort study. Prasad and colleagues[6] compared 132 patients treated endoscopically with 46 patients treated with esophagectomy. In the endoscopically treated group, 57% of the patients received ER alone and 43% had a combination of ER and PDT. The endoscopically treated group and the surgery group differed significantly with regard to age, length of the Barrett's segment, and comorbidity. The recurrence rates were 12% in the endoscopic group and 2% in the surgery group. The overall survival rates were comparable in the two groups, but cancer-free survival was superior in the surgery group.

ER in Submucosal Cancer

Whether cancers limited to the upper submucosal layer (sm1) are eligible for ER in selected cases is not as yet clear. Surgical series have been able to show that patients with sm1 Barrett's cancer have a very low risk of metastatic lymph nodes, but larger series reporting on the endoscopic treatment of these patients are still lacking. A recently published series from the authors' department could demonstrate that ER seems to be safe also in patients with low-risk submucosal cancer (T1sm1, G1-2, L0, V0, macroscopic type I or II): 21 patients were treated by ER.[26] One patient was referred to surgery and one patient died (not tumor-related) before complete remission could be achieved. A total of 18 out of 19 patients achieved complete remission after a mean of 2.9 ER and 5.3 months. After a mean follow-up of 62 months recurrent or metachronous neoplasia was detected in five patients, but repeat endoscopic treatment was successful in all of these patients. The calculated 5-year over-all survival rate was 66%. However, no tumor-related death occurred in this series.

Those promising results suggest that ER also could be successful in low-risk sm1 Barrett's cancer in a highly experienced center, but further data have to be awaited to draw final conclusions. Patients with deep submucosal invasion (sm2–3 or invasion >500 μm) should be treated by esophagectomy, whenever possible, because lymph node risk is up to 40% in these patients.

SUMMARY

ER is the ideal treatment for early neoplastic lesions in Barrett's esophagus. It combines effective treatment of neoplasia limited to the mucosal layer with the ability of an exact histologic diagnosis of the infiltration depth of the tumor and whether it is infiltrating lymph or blood vessels. Many studies from different centers were able to demonstrate that ER is safe in expert hands and highly effective going along with a complete remission rate of usually more than 95%. The problem of the relatively high rate of recurrences and metachronous neoplasia seems to be solved by a combination of ER with ablative treatment (eg, with APC or RFA) of the remaining nondysplastic Barrett's esophagus.

REFERENCES

1. Pech O, May A, Rabenstein T, et al. Endoscopic resection of early oesophageal cancer. Gut 2007;56:1625–34.
2. Buskens CJ, Westerterp M, Lagarde SM, et al. Prediction of appropriateness of local endoscopic treatment for high-grade dysplasia and early adenocarcinoma by EUS and histopathologic features. Gastrointest Endosc 2004;60: 703–10.
3. Stein HJ, Feith M, Bruecher BLDM, et al. Early esophageal squamous cell and adenocarcinoma: pattern of lymphatic spread and prognostic factors for long term survival after surgical resection. Ann Surg 2005;242:566–73.
4. Rice TW, Blackstone EH, Goldblum JR, et al. Superficial adenocarcinoma of the esophagus. J Thorac Cardiovasc Surg 2001;122:1077–90.
5. Oh DS, Hagen JA, Chandrasoma PT, et al. Clinical biology and surgical therapy of intramucosal adenocarcinoma of the esophagus. J Am Coll Surg 2006;203: 152–61.
6. Prasad GA, Wu TT, Wigle DA, et al. Endoscopic and surgical treatment of mucosal (T1a) esophageal adenocarcinoma in Barrett's esophagus. Gastroenterology 2009;137:815–23.
7. Pech O, May A, Günter E, et al. The impact of endoscopic ultrasound and computed tomography on the TNM staging of early cancer in Barrett's esophagus. Am J Gastroenterol 2006;101:2223–9.
8. Chemaly M, Scalone O, Durivage G, et al. Miniprobe EUS in the pretherapeutic assessment of early esophageal neoplasia. Endoscopy 2008;40(1):2–6.
9. Rampado S, Bocus P, Battaglia G, et al. Endoscopic ultrasound: accuracy in staging superficial carcinomas of the esophagus. Ann Thorac Surg 2008;85(1): 251–26.
10. Pech O, Günter E, Dusemund F, et al. Value of high-frequency miniprobes and conventional radial endoscopic ultrasound in the staging of early Barrett's carcinoma. Endoscopy 2010;42(2):98–103.
11. Pech O, Günter E, Dusemund F, et al. Accuracy of endoscopic ultrasound in preoperative staging of esophageal cancer: results from a referral center for early esophageal cancer. Endoscopy 2010;42(6):456–61.

12. Inoue H, Endo M. A new simplified technique of endoscopic esophageal mucosal resection using a cap-fitted panendoscope. Surg Endosc 1993;6: 264–5.
13. May A, Gossner L, Behrens A, et al. A prospective randomized trial of two different suck-and-cut mucosectomy techniques in 100 consecutive resections in patients with early cancer of the esophagus. Gastrointest Endosc 2003;58: 167–75.
14. Peters FP, Kara MA, Curvers WL, et al. Multiband mucosectomy for endoscopic resection of Barrett's esophagus: feasibility study with matched historical controls. Eur J Gastroenterol Hepatol 2007;19(4):311–5.
15. Hosokawa K, Yoshida S. [Recent advances in endoscopic mucosal resection for early gastric cancer]. Gan To Kagaku Ryoho 1998;25:476–83 [in Japanese].
16. Ono H, Kondo H, Gotoda T, et al. Endoscopic mucosal resection for treatment of early gastric cancer. Gut 2001;48:225–9.
17. Ell C, May A, Gossner L, et al. Endoscopic mucosal resection of early cancer and high-grade dysplasia in Barrett's esophagus. Gastroenterology 2000;118(4): 670–7.
18. Ell C, May A, Pech O, et al. Curative endoscopic resection of early esophageal adenocarcinomas (Barrett's cancer). Gastrointest Endosc 2007;65:3–10.
19. Pech O, Behrens A, May A, et al. Long-term results and risk factor analysis for recurrence after curative endoscopic therapy in 349 patients with high-grade intraepithelial neoplasia and mucosal adenocarcinoma in Barrett's oesophagus. Gut 2008;57:1200–6.
20. Peters FP, Kara MA, Rosmolen WD, et al. Stepwise radical endoscopic resection is effective for complete removal of Barrett's esophagus with early neoplasia: a prospective study. Am J Gastroenterol 2006;101:1449–157.
21. Chennat J, Konda VJA, Ross AS, et al. Complete Barrett's eradication endoscopic mucosal resection (CBE-EMR): an effective treatment modality for high grade dysplasia (HGD) and intramucosal carcinoma (IMC). An American single center experience. Am J Gastroenterol 2009;104(11): 2684–292.
22. Pouw RE, Wirths K, Eisendrath P, et al. Efficacy of radiofrequency ablation combined with endoscopic resection for Barrett's esophagus with early neoplasia. Clin Gastroenterol Hepatol 2010;8(1):23–9.
23. Pouw RE, Seewald S, Gondrie JJ, et al. Stepwise radical endoscopic resection for eradication of Barrett's oesophagus with early neoplasia in a cohort of 169 patients. Gut 2010;59(9):1169–77.
24. Bollschweiler E, Baldus SE, Schröder W, et al. High rate of lymph-node metastasis in submucosal esophageal squamous-cell carcinomas and adenocarcinomas. Endoscopy 2006;38:149–56.
25. Ancona E, Rampado S, Cassaro M, et al. Prediction of lymph node status in superficial esophageal carcinoma. Ann Surg Oncol 2008;15(11):3278–88.
26. Manner H, May A, Pech O, et al. Early Barrett's carcinoma with "low-risk" submucosal invasion: long-term results of endoscopic resection with a curative intent. Am J Gastroenterol 2008;103(10):2589–297.
27. Badreddine RJ, Prasad GA, Lewis JT, et al. Depth of submucosal invasion does not predict lymph node metastasis and survival of patients with esophageal carcinoma. Clin Gastroenterol Hepatol 2010;8(3):248–53.
28. May A, Gossner L, Pech O, et al. Local endoscopic therapy for intraepithelial high-grade neoplasia and early adenocarcinoma in Barrett's oesophagus: acute-phase

and intermediate results of a new treatment approach. Eur J Gastroenterol Hepatol 2002;14(10):1085–91.

29. Manner H, Rabenstein T, Braun K, et al. What should we do with the remainder of the Barrett's segment after endoscopic resection of early Barrett's cancer? Intermediate results of the first prospective-randomized trial on the APC ablation of residual Barrett's mucosa with concomitant esomeprazole therapy versus surveillance without ablation after ER of early Barrett's cancer. Gastrointest Endosc 2010;71(5):AB175.

30. Gondrie JJ, Pouw RE, Sondermeijer C, et al. Effective treatment of early Barrett's neoplasia with stepwise circumferential and focal ablation using the HALO system. Endoscopy 2008;40:370–39.

31. Gondrie JJ, Pouw RE, Sondermeijer C, et al. Stepwise circumferential and focal ablation of Barrett's esophagus with high-grade dysplasia: results of the first prospective series in 11 patients. Endoscopy 2008;40:359–69.

32. Pech O, Gossner L, Manner H, et al. Prospective evaluation of the macroscopic types and location of early Barrett's neoplasia in 380 lesions. Endoscopy 2007;39:588–93.

33. Peters FP, Brakenhoff KP, Curvers WL, et al. Histologic evaluation of resection specimens obtained at 293 endoscopic resections in Barrett's esophagus. Gastrointest Endosc 2008;67:604–9.

34. Seewald S, Akaraviputh T, Seitz U, et al. Circumferential EMR and complete removal of Barrett's epithelium: a new approach to management of Barrett's esophagus containing high-grade intraepithelial neoplasia and intramucosal carcinoma. Gastrointest Endosc 2003;57:854–9.

35. Giovannini M, Bories E, Pesenti C, et al. Circumferential endoscopic mucosal resection in Barrett's esophagus with high-grade intraepithelial neoplasia or mucosal cancer: preliminary results in 21 patients. Endoscopy 2004;36:782–7.

36. Soehendra N, Seewald S, Groth S, et al. Use of modified multiband ligator facilitates circumferential EMR in Barrett's esophagus (with video). Gastrointest Endosc 2006;63:847–52.

37. Larghi A, Lightdale CJ, Ross AS, et al. Long-term follow-up of complete Barrett's eradication endoscopic mucosal resection (CBE-EMR) for the treatment of high grade dysplasia and intramucosal carcinoma. Endoscopy 2007;39(12):1086–91.

38. Lopes CV, Hela M, Pesenti C, et al. Circumferential endoscopic resection of Barrett's esophagus with high-grade dysplasia or early adenocarcinoma. Surg Endosc 2007;21(5):820–4.

39. Kakushima N, Yahagi N, Fujishiro M, et al. Efficacy and safety of endoscopic submucosal dissection for tumors of the esophagogastric junction. Endoscopy 2006;38:170–4.

40. Yoshinaga S, Gotoda T, Kusano C, et al. Clinical impact of endoscopic submucosal dissection for superficial adenocarcinoma located at the esophagogastric junction. Gastrointest Endosc 2008;67(2):202–9.

41. Deprez PH, Piessevaux H, Aouattah T, et al. ESD in Barrett's esophagus high grade dysplasia and mucosal cancer: prospective comparison with CAP mucosectomy. Gastrointest Endosc 2010;71(5):AB126.

42. Nijhawan PK, Wang KK. Endoscopic mucosal resection for lesions with endoscopic features suggestive of malignancy and high-grade dysplasia within Barrett's esophagus. Gastrointest Endosc 2000;52:328–32.

43. Buttar NS, Wang KK, Lutzke LS, et al. Combined endoscopic mucosal resection and photodynamic therapy for esophageal neoplasia within Barrett's esophagus. Gastrointest Endosc 2001;54:682–8.
44. Behrens A, May A, Gossner L, et al. Curative treatment for high-grade intraepithelial neoplasia in Barrett's esophagus. Endoscopy 2005;37:999–1005.
45. Conio M, Repici A, Cestari R, et al. Endoscopic mucosal resection for high-grade dysplasia and intramucosal carcinoma in Barrett's esophagus: an Italian experience. World J Gastroenterol 2005;11:6650–5.
46. Thomas T, Singh R, Ragunath K. Trimodal imaging-assisted endoscopic mucosal resection of early Barrett's neoplasia. Surg Endosc 2009;23:1609–13.
47. Pech O, Manner H, May A, et al. Endoscopic therapy in 1059 patients with high grade dysplasia and early adenocarcinoma in Barrett's esophagus: lessons we have learned. Gastrointest Endosc 2009;69(5):AB114–AB5.

The Role of Radiofrequency Ablation in the Management of Barrett's Esophagus

William J. Bulsiewicz, MD, MSc[a], Nicholas J. Shaheen, MD, MPH[b],*

KEYWORDS

- Radiofrequency ablation • Barrett's esophagus
- Dysplasia • Intestinal metaplasia

Despite the presence of Barrett's esophagus (BE) in 1% to 2% of the US population, its association with progression to esophageal adenocarcinoma, and a 500% increase in the incidence of esophageal adenocarcinoma (EAC) since the 1970s, the optimal management strategy for BE has not been clearly defined.[1,2] When BE does progress, it seems to do so through a series of morphologic changes, from low-grade dysplasia (LGD), to high-grade dysplasia (HGD), and on to cancer. Given the 5-year survival rate of 13% for esophageal adenocarcinoma, 3 treatment strategies have been used for patients with BE and HGD: esophagectomy, intensive endoscopic surveillance, and mucosal eradication.[3–7] Although usually curative, esophagectomy is associated with 3% to 5% mortality, 40% to 50% morbidity, and permanent loss of esophageal function.[8] Meanwhile, intensive endoscopic surveillance is time and resource intensive, and still has a risk of disease progression to EAC as high as 19% at 1 year and 50% at 3 years.[9,10]

Given the shortcomings of the competing strategies, mucosal ablation is appealing as a potential treatment strategy for dysplastic BE. Among the multiple endoscopic ablative strategies that have been studied in recent years, radiofrequency ablation (RFA) has shown promise because 2 prospective, multicenter clinical trials have shown it to be effective, safe, and well-tolerated.[9,11] Further data are accumulating to determine whether RFA is durable and cost-effective.

[a] GI Outcomes Training Program, University of North Carolina School of Medicine, Chapel Hill, NC, USA
[b] Division of Gastroenterology, Center for Esophageal Diseases and Swallowing, University of North Carolina School of Medicine, CB#7080, Chapel Hill, NC 27599–7080, USA
* Corresponding author.
E-mail address: nshaheen@med.unc.edu

Gastrointest Endoscopy Clin N Am 21 (2011) 95–109
doi:10.1016/j.giec.2010.09.009
1052-5157/11/$ – see front matter © 2011 Elsevier Inc. All rights reserved.

This article reviews the evidence behind RFA to differentiate it from other management strategies in terms of efficacy, durability, safety, tolerability, and cost-effectiveness. The role of RFA in the management of BE is described, including endoscopic resection. Future directions are identified for research that will help to better define the role of RFA in the management of BE.

WHAT IS RADIOFREQUENCY ABLATION?
Principles of RFA

In RFA, an alternating electrical current induces an electromagnetic field causing charged ions to rapidly oscillate, collide with one another, and create molecular friction that results in a rapid, exothermic release of thermal energy. Applied directly to esophageal tissue, it allows controlled thermal injury leading to water vaporization, coagulation of proteins, and cell necrosis. One significant advantage of RFA compared with other ablative modalities is that desiccated tissue has a much higher resistance to current than normal tissue. Thus, the coagulated lipids and proteins act as an insulator such that the system delivers an ablation depth that is consistent and well-controlled, dependent on the energy output of the probe and the frequency of the current.[12,13] Seamless contact between the esophagus and the ablation interface is necessary for effective mucosal eradication to occur, and the device provides a superficial depth of injury. Therefore, RFA should generally not be applied to nodular tissue with curative intent.

Device and Procedural Technique

The only commercially available RFA system (BÂRRX Medical, Inc, Sunnyvale, CA, USA) consists of 2 partner devices, the HALO[360] device and HALO[90] device, which perform circumferential and focal ablation, respectively. The HALO[360] system consists of a sizing balloon, a balloon-based ablation catheter, and an energy generator. The ablation catheter contains a microelectrode array encircling a balloon that is capable of delivering radiofrequency energy. The array consists of 60 tightly spaced bipolar electrodes circumferentially surrounding the balloon and covering a total length of 3-cm of the balloon. The energy generator provides automated, pressure-regulated air inflation of the sizing balloon and ablation catheters. During ablation, it rapidly delivers a preset density of radiofrequency energy, measured in joules per cm^2, to the catheter electrode.

To perform circumferential ablation, an upper endoscopy is first performed, and the length of BE is measured (**Fig. 1**A). Next, a sizing balloon is used to measure the inner diameter of the esophagus with a pressure/volume algorithm. The ablation catheter is selected such that the outer diameter of the balloon approximates the measured inner diameter of the esophagus, and then introduced over a guidewire, followed by the endoscope above it. Using endoscopic guidance, the proximal-most electrode is positioned 1 cm above the proximal edge of the BE and, by a single depression of a foot pedal, the device is activated to inflate the balloon and deliver the prespecified energy. After the first ablation, the endoscopist deflates the balloon and advances the catheter distally such that the proximal-most electrode is now aligned with the distal ablation zone, with minimal overlap (see **Fig. 1**B). Ablation is again performed, and this sequence is continued until the ablation zone extends to the top of the gastric folds. At this point, the endoscope and the ablation balloon are removed from the patient. Coagulative debris are removed from the surface of the balloon using a damp 4×4-cm gauze. A soft plastic cap is affixed to the endoscope, and the patient is reintubated with the endoscope. Using the end of the cap, and with copious lavage,

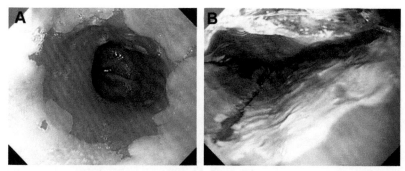

Fig. 1. Circumferential RFA in the treatment of Barrett's esophagus. (A) The distal esophagus of a patient with Barrett's metaplasia before ablation. The pale mucosa in the foreground is normal squamous epithelium, whereas the salmon-colored tissue distally is Barrett's epithelium. (B) The coagulative effect of an application of the HALO[360] device. The HALO[360] device is seen at 12 o'clock with the balloon deflated.

the treated area is debrided to remove all coagulative debris and prepare the area for a second treatment. Based on phase 2 studies using the RFA device and examining efficacy, a second treatment is then performed in similar fashion through the entire ablation zone.[14]

The HALO[90] system consists of a device that fits on the tip of the gastroscope and is connected to the HALO[360] energy generator. The upper surface of the device has an articulated platform measuring 20-mm long by 13-mm wide with an electrode array, arranged in a similar fashion to the circumferential device. During focal ablation, the electrode is positioned on the target tissue, and then the endoscope tip is deflected up, bringing the electrode into contact with the esophageal tissue (**Fig. 2**A). Energy is delivered twice to this area (see **Fig. 2**B). Afterward, the rounded, distal-most edge of the ablation catheter is used to clean coagulum from the ablation zone. The endoscope and attached device are then removed from the esophagus and cleaned. After cleaning, the endoscope and device are reinserted into the esophagus and energy again applied to the target area an additional 2 times, bringing the total number of applications to 4 per targeted area in the esophagus (see **Fig. 2**C).

Ablation procedures may be performed in the outpatient setting using conscious sedation. The median time to complete the procedure is roughly 30 minutes for a circumferential procedure and 20 minutes for a focal procedure.[9,11] Barring unforeseen complications, patients return home the same day and do not require inpatient admission. Oral analgesics are usually given to be used as needed for periprocedural discomfort.

EFFICACY, DURABILITY, AND COST-EFFECTIVENESS OF RFA
In High-grade Dysplastic BE

As shown in **Table 1**, there have been 9 published studies to date that have analyzed the efficacy of RFA for HGD.[9,15–23] Among 237 patients with HGD followed for a mean of 13.3 months, complete remission of intestinal metaplasia (CRIM) was noted in 67%, whereas complete remission of dysplasia (CRD) was noted in 84%.

CRIM after RFA ranged from 54% (92 patients at 12 months) to 100% (11 patients at 14 months).[19,21] The cohort of 92 patients studied by Ganz and colleagues[19] also happened to be the largest analysis of patients with HGD. However, patients in this nonrandomized, retrospective study without a control arm received a mean of just

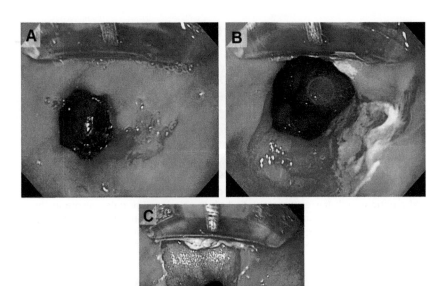

Fig. 2. Focal RFA in the treatment of Barrett's esophagus. (*A*) The distal esophagus with a short segment of Barrett epithelium at 4 o'clock. The HALO[90] device is seen at 12 o'clock, in contact with esophageal mucosa before focal ablation. (*B*) Radiofrequency energy being applied for the first time using the HALO[90] device to the esophageal mucosa at 12 o'clock. At 4 o'clock is a rectangular area of white coagulum immediately after focal RFA. (*C*) The distal esophagus after 2 rounds of focal ablation. In the treatment zones at 12 o'clock and 6 o'clock, the coagulum has been debrided. The HALO[90] device is positioned at 12 o'clock.

1.6 ablations. Of all studies ablating HGD, this was the smallest number of ablations, with the largest being 4.0.

CRD ranged from 79% (24 patients at 21 months) to 100% (11 patients at 14 months).[21,24] In the study by Ganz and colleagues,[19] again the largest cohort of patients with HGD, CRD was achieved in 80% at 12 months with just 1.6 ablations.

In considering the efficacy of RFA in the treatment of HGD, special attention should be given to the AIM Dysplasia trial; a prospective, multicenter, sham-controlled trial of RFA to treat BE.[9] In this study, 127 patients with dysplasia were randomized in a 2:1 ratio to receive either RFA or a sham procedure. Randomization was stratified according to the grade of dysplasia and the length of intestinal metaplasia. All patients received intensive endoscopic surveillance. The primary outcomes of interest were the CRD or the CRIM, both assessed at 12 months following initial intervention. Secondary outcomes of interest included an assessment of progression of dysplasia as well as the number of biopsies free of intestinal metaplasia at 12 months. An intention-to-treat analysis (ITT) was performed in addition to analysis per-protocol.

The results of the study showed RFA to be an effective treatment strategy for the eradication of metaplasia and dysplasia, compared with the control group. At 12 months and after a mean of 3.5 ablation treatments per patient, 83% achieved CRIM (77% ITT), whereas 92% achieved CRD (86% ITT). Among the control patients

Table 1
Efficacy and durability of RFA for BE

First Author	Year	All Patients Studied — No. Patients	Ave. Follow-up (mo)	CRIM (%)	CRD (%)	HGD Subgroup — No. Patients	CRIM (%)	CRD (%)	LGD Subgroup — No. Patients	CRIM (%)	CRD (%)	NDBE Subgroup — No. Patients	CRIM (%)
Lyday et al[15]	2010	338	9	72	89	31	55	83	42	71	95	265	75
—		137	20	77	100	10	80	100	13	85	100	114	76
Vassiliou et al[16]	2010	14	20	79	NA	10	80	NA	2	100	100	1	100
Pouw et al[17]	2010	24	22	88	95	10	NA	NA	11	NA	NA	3	NA
Sharma et al[24]	2009	63	21	79	89	24	67	79	39	79	89	0	NA
Velanovich[18]	2009	66	12	93	NA	7	100	100	NA	NA	NA	NA	NA
Shaheen et al[9]	2009	84	12	77	86	42	74	81	42	81	90	0	NA
Eldaif et al[28]	2009	27	2	100	100	0	NA	NA	2	100	100	25	100
Ganz et al[19]	2008	92	12	54	80	92	54	80	0	NA	NA	0	NA
Gondrie et al[20]	2008	11	14	100	100	9	100	100	2	100	100	0	NA
Fleischer et al[11]	2008	62	30	97	NA	0	NA	NA	0	NA	NA	62	97
Hernandez et al[22]	2008	10	12	70	NA	1	100	100	2	100	100	7	57
Sharma et al[29]	2008	10	24	90	100	0	NA	NA	10	90	100	0	NA
Gondrie et al[21]	2008	12	14	100	100	11	100	100	1	100	100	0	NA
Sharma et al[30]	2007	100	12	67	NA	0	NA	NA	0	NA	NA	100	67
Roorda et al[23]	2007	13	12	46	71	3	NA	NA	4	NA	NA	6	NA
Aggregate data		**1063**	**14**	**76**	**90**	**237**	**67**	**84**	**155**	**80**	**93**	**574**	**77**

Abbreviations: CRIM, complete remission of intestinal metaplasia; CRD, complete remission of dysplasia; NA, not applicable; NDBE, nondysplastic BE.

who received a sham procedure and high-dose proton pump inhibitory therapy, 3% achieved CRIM and 23% achieved CRD. In both the CRIM and CRD analyses, the results showed a statistically significant difference between the treatment and control groups (P<.001 in both cases). Only 4% of the treatment arm had disease progression, compared with 16% among the control group (P = .03). Among biopsies taken at 12 months, 98% of those taken in the treatment group were free of intestinal metaplasia, versus 58% in the control group (P<.001).

Specific to HGD, the randomized controlled trial noted CRIM among 82% (74% ITT) and CRD among 90% (81% ITT). In comparison with the rates noted in the control group (0% CRIM, 19% CRD), the differences between the groups were statistically significant (P<.001 in both cases). Disease progression to cancer occurred in 2.4% of the treatment group and 19.0% of the control group, also a statistically significant difference (P = .04). Among biopsies taken at 12 months, 98% of those taken in the treatment group were free of intestinal metaplasia, versus 59% in the control group (P<.001).

In terms of durability, the longest study in manuscript form to date to analyze RFA in HGD among more than 10 patients was published by Sharma and colleagues.[24] Using a protocol of stepwise progressive ablation until complete remission of intestinal metaplasia was achieved, 67% CRIM and 79% CRD was noted among 24 patients with HGD after a median of 18 months of observation. The short duration of this study shows the need for further, long-term studies of RFA in HGD to adequately determine its durability. Recently, longer-term follow-up of the subjects from the randomized controlled trial was presented in abstract form.[25] These data suggest that the reversion attained in the treatment phase of the study is durable at the 2- to 3-year follow-up time point.

In comparison with other modalities of ablation, RFA has shown comparable, if not superior, efficacy. In a multicenter, randomized trial comparing photodynamic therapy (PDT) with surveillance, PDT achieved CRD in 77% of patients with HGD at 18 months.[10] However, 13% who received PDT progressed to esophageal cancer at 18 months. In a recent nonrandomized, retrospective analysis of 60 patients with HGD undergoing a mean of 4.0 cryoablation treatments, 87% achieved CRD and 57% achieved CRIM after an average of 10.5 months.[26] Whether this technology will emerge as an alternative to RFA therapy is unclear given the preliminary nature of the data. Overall, current data suggest that RFA is as or more effective than other commonly used modalities of ablation.

In a cost-effectiveness analysis of ablative strategies published before the AIM Dysplasia trial, RFA seems to be a cost-effective strategy.[27] Compared with argon plasma coagulation (APC), RFA was more effective and less costly, and therefore the dominant treatment strategy. Compared with PDT, RFA was similarly effective and much less costly. PDT was associated with an incremental cost-effectiveness ratio of more than $32 million per discounted quality-adjusted life year (dQALY), when compared with treatment with RFA. Based on this, sensitivity analyses showed that RFA would be the most cost-effective strategy if less than 18% had residual HGD after RFA. Given the results of the AIM Dysplasia trial, in which 90% with HGD achieved CRD, RFA seems to be a more cost-effective strategy than PDT. This analysis assumes that regression of metaplasia is durable, a contention which is unproven. Therefore, this analysis will need to be revisited when durability data of the modalities are clarified. Cryotherapy was not included in this analysis, and will need to be considered in future analyses of cost-effectiveness.

In considering RFA against nonablative management of HGD, several advantages exist for RFA. First, intensive endoscopic surveillance bears up to a 19% risk of progression to esophageal adenocarcinoma at 1 year, and 50% at 3 years.[9,10] This risk can be significantly reduced using RFA, as shown by the AIM Dysplasia trial. Second, RFA has an excellent safety profile, as shown in **Table 2** and detailed later, in particular when compared with the mortality and morbidity associated with esophagectomy.[8] Other advantages of RFA compared with esophagectomy include that RFA is an outpatient same-day procedure, and that RFA does not irreversibly alter the esophageal anatomy. Also, if RFA fails to eliminate dysplasia, surgery remains an option for the future. Ablation by any modality seems less costly and also more effective than either endoscopic surveillance or immediate esophagectomy.[27]

Thus, RFA has shown adequate efficacy and cost-effectiveness to be considered as a first-line option for HGD. Further studies are necessary to determine the durability of RFA for HGD, which will help to clarify postablation surveillance protocols and further clarify the cost-effectiveness of RFA compared with surveillance, surgery, and other ablation modalities.

In Low-grade Dysplastic BE

As shown in **Table 1**, there have been 9 published studies to date that have analyzed the efficacy of RFA for LGD.[9,15–23] Among 155 patients with LGD followed for a mean of 14.9 months, CRIM was noted in 80%, whereas CRD was noted in 93%.

CRIM after RFA ranged from 71% (42 patients at 9 months) to 90% among 10 patients at 24 months or 100% among 2 patients in several studies.[15,16,20,22,28,29] The study of 42 patients published by Lyday and colleagues[15] is unique in that it contains the only data examining the efficacy of RFA among community-based gastroenterologists. This study was a multicenter registry conducted at 4 community-based practices, with varying study methods among the 4 sites. These data were obtained after 1.8 ablations, which is on the low end of the range between 1.1 and 4.0, with the median number of ablations being 2.5 per patient. CRD ranged from 89% (39 patients at 21 months) to 100% (13 patients at 20 months).[15,24]

In considering the efficacy of RFA in the treatment of LGD, the[9] AIM Dysplasia trial studied the largest cohort of patients with LGD (42, tied with Lyday and colleagues). Among patients with LGD, 85% achieved CRIM (81% ITT) and 95% achieved CRD (ITT 90%). In comparison with the rates noted in the control group (4% CRIM, 23% CRD), the differences between the groups were statistically significant ($P<.001$ in both cases). Disease progression to cancer occurred in no patients in either the treatment or control group. Meanwhile, progression from LGD to HGD occurred in 4.8% of the treatment group and 13.6% of the control group, which was not a statistically significant difference ($P = .33$). Among biopsies taken at 12 months, 98% of those taken in the treatment group were free of intestinal metaplasia, versus 57% in the control group ($P<.001$).

In terms of durability, the longest study to date to analyze RFA in LGD among more than 10 patients was published by Sharma and colleagues.[24] As previously described, using a protocol of stepwise progressive ablation until complete remission of intestinal metaplasia was achieved, 79% CRIM and 89% CRD was noted among 39 patients with LGD after a median of 23 months of observation. Again, long-term studies are necessary to adequately determine the durability of RFA in LGD.

In considering RFA against alternative strategies for LGD, RFA seems to be a cost-effective strategy.[27] When compared with intensive endoscopic surveillance, RFA was more effective and less costly, and therefore the dominant option. In sensitivity analysis, if less than 46% of patients had CRD after ablation, surveillance became the more cost-effective strategy. As shown by the results in **Table 1**, RFA has consistently shown the ability to induce remission of dysplasia in more than

Table 2
Safety and tolerability of RFA for BE

First Author	Year	No. Patients	Ave. Follow-up (mo)	Mean Treatments	Perforations (%)	Strictures	Subsquamous Metaplasia (%)	Bleeding (%)	Hospitalizations (%)	Chest Pain or Dysphagia (%)	Nausea (%)
Lyday et al[15]	2010	429	12	1.8	0 (0)	9 (2)	0 (0)	5 (1)	0 (0)	NA	NA
Vassiliou et al[16]	2010	25	20	2.4	0 (0)	2 (8)	0 (0)	1 (4)	0 (0)	0 (0)	2 (8)
Pouw et al[17]	2010	24	22	3.0	1 (4)a	1 (4)	0 (0)	1 (4)	0 (0)	NA	NA
Sharma et al[24]	2009	63	21	NA	0 (0)	1 (2)	0 (0)	1 (2)	0 (0)	NA	NA
Velanovich[18]	2009	66	12	NA	0 (0)	4 (6)	NA	0 (0)	0 (0)	NA	NA
Shaheen et al[9]	2009	78	12	3.5	0 (0)	5 (6)	4 (5)	1 (1)	2 (2)	2 (2)	1 (1)
Eldaif et al[28]	2009	27	2	1.1	0 (0)	0 (0)	0 (0)	0 (0)	0 (0)	0 (0)	0 (0)
Ganz et al[19]	2008	142	12	1.6	0 (0)	1 (1)	0 (0)	NA	NA	NA	NA
Gondrie et al[20]	2008	11	14	3.0	0 (0)	0 (0)	0 (0)	0 (0)	0 (0)	NA	NA
Fleischer et al[11]	2008	62	30	3.4	0 (0)	0 (0)	0 (0)	1 (1)	0 (0)	10 (16)	10 (16)
Hernandez et al[22]	2008	10	12	1.8	0 (0)	0 (0)	1 (10)	0 (0)	0 (0)	NA	NA
Sharma et al[29]	2008	10	24	2.5	0 (0)	0 (0)	0 (0)	1 (10)	1 (10)	NA	NA
Gondrie et al[21]	2008	12	14	4.0	0 (0)	1 (8)	0 (0)	0 (0)	0 (0)	NA	NA
Sharma et al[30]	2007	100	12	1.5	0 (0)	0 (0)	0 (0)	1 (1)	0 (0)	12 (12)	9 (9)
Roorda et al[23]	2007	13	12	1.4	0 (0)	0 (0)	0 (0)	0 (0)	0 (0)	3 (23)	NA
Aggregate data		**1072**	**14**	**2.1**	**0.1a**	**2.2**	**0.5**	**1.3**	**0.3**	**8.9**	**7.5**

Abbreviation: NA, not applicable.
a Occurred after endoscopic mucosal resection. There are no reports of perforation with an intact mucosa and muscularis before RFA.

90% of patients, far surpassing the necessary efficacy to be cost-effective. When compared with APC and PDT, RFA was similarly effective and less costly, particularly when compared with PDT. Again, this study was published before the results of the AIM Dysplasia trial. Thus, the most cost-effective strategy is likely RFA with further surveillance limited to those who have residual metaplasia on follow-up biopsies. A strategy of no intervention with no surveillance, although cost-effective, carries significant risk because it is impossible to predict which patients will progress to HGD or EAC. Per 100 patients with LGD, approximately 10 fewer cancers are predicted to develop if ablation is performed, as opposed to no further surveillance.[27]

Thus, RFA seems to possess adequate efficacy and cost-effectiveness to be considered as a potential therapy for selected patients with low-grade dysplastic BE, in particular because it is impossible to predict who will advance to HGD or EAC, or when this will happen. Further studies are necessary to better determine the natural history of LGD and the durability of RFA for LGD, which, as in HGD, will help to clarify postablation surveillance protocols and further clarify the cost-effectiveness of RFA compared with alternative options. When considering RFA in patients with LGD, it is important to discuss with them the lack of direct evidence of a decreased cancer risk with RFA, and the good prognosis of LGD without intervention. Even with these caveats, ablation may be attractive, especially to the young patient, the patient with multifocal LGD, and the patient with LGD on several biopsy sessions.

In Nondysplastic BE

As shown in **Table 1**, there have been 6 published studies to date that have analyzed the efficacy of RFA for nondysplastic Barrett's esophagus (NDBE).[11,15,17,22,28,30] Among 574 patients with NDBE followed for a mean of 13.7 months, CRIM was noted in 77%. The range for CRIM after RFA was 57% (7 patients at 12 months) to 100% (25 patients at 2 months).[22,28]

In considering the efficacy of RFA in the treatment of NDBE, special attention should be given to the prospective, multicenter study of RFA in NDBE by Fleischer and colleagues[11] and Sharma and colleagues.[30] Seventy patients were enrolled at 8 US medical centers with between 2 and 6 cm of NDBE. Each participant received circumferential ablation at baseline. Follow-up biopsies were obtained at 1, 3, 6, 12, and 30 months. If residual intestinal metaplasia was identified at 1 or 3 months, repeat circumferential ablation was performed at 4 months. At 12 months, focal ablation was performed if either histologic or gross evidence of residual BE was identified. The primary outcome of interest was the complete remission of intestinal metaplasia, assessed at 12 and 30 months. The incidence of adverse events was also monitored.

At 12 months, CRIM was achieved among 70% of 69 patients after undergoing a mean of 1.5 circumferential ablation treatments.[30] Sixty-two of the 70 patients agreed to continue in the trial. After a mean of 1.9 focal ablation procedures, CRIM was achieved in 98% of 61 patients at 30 months.[11] Thus, the combination of circumferential and focal RFA for NDBE showed excellent efficacy with durability out to 30 months. However, the 30 months includes the time that ablation procedures are being performed. Further studies are necessary to determine the durability of RFA from the time CRIM is achieved and no further ablation procedures are necessary.

In terms of cost-effectiveness, RFA with surveillance limited to those with residual metaplasia seems to be the most cost-effective approach.[27] Strategies that use surveillance followed by ablation if progression to dysplasia, or ablation followed by continued surveillance, are dominated by this model. Again, there are only data on the durability of intestinal metaplasia to 30 months. However, in sensitivity analysis, there would need to be permanent eradication of metaplasia in 47% or more to make surveillance a more cost-effective strategy. Given that 97% had eradication of intestinal metaplasia at 30 months in the study by Fleischer and colleagues,[11] short- to midterm results suggest that RFA may have the durability necessary to be cost-effective.

In considering treatment strategies for NDBE, the absolute risk of progression to cancer may be low enough to favor a strategy of no intervention and no surveillance. However, the cumulative likelihood of disease progression increases as time passes. After a mean of 4.2 years of follow-up among 618 patients with NDBE, Sharma and colleagues[31] reported a total rate of progression of 21.7%. Most of these were to LGD (16.2%), but some patients advanced to either HGD (3.6%) or esophageal adeno-carcinoma (2.0%). At 8 years, 5% of the cohort had progressed to EAC (0.6% per patient year of follow-up). Therefore, there may be a subgroup of patients with NDBE in whom ablation is a reasonable alternative. Again, the issue of inadequate risk strat-ification is present; although targeting young patients with NDBE seems obvious, given their larger cumulative risk, even among these patients, most will not progress to cancer, and therefore would not benefit from therapy. Individual treatment decisions will be based on patient and physician preferences, and should recognize the lack of data substantiating a reduced risk of cancer after ablation in the population of patients with NDBE. Also, although the safety profile of RFA is excellent, no data exist to deter-mine whether RFA has the durability to last 5, 10 or more years after ablation without disease recurrence. Ideally, long-term studies and better predictive models would help in determining the best course of action, as well as the appropriate surveillance protocol following ablation. Until patients who will progress to worse disease can be better identify from the large pool of patients with NDBE, a broad recommendation in favor of ablative therapy in all patients with NDBE cannot be made.

PATIENT SAFETY AND TOLERABILITY OF RFA

As shown in **Table 2**, all 15 studies that reported efficacy data (shown in **Table 1**) have also reported data on safety outcomes. Through all 15 studies, 1072 patients have undergone an average of 2.1 ablations each. Among the more than 2000 ablations performed there is only 1 report of esophageal perforation.[17] Of note, the single report of esophageal perforation occurred in a patient after endoscopic mucosal resection and before RFA had been performed. Thus, there are no reports to date of perforation following RFA. Nevertheless, excluding the 2 studies that did not include data on the number of treatments received by patients, the risk of esophageal perforation can conservatively be estimated at less than 1:1950 treatments received.

In similar fashion, the rate of strictures compares favorably with other modes of ablation. In total among the 15 studies, 2.2% of patients reported strictures. By excluding the 2 studies that did not report the number of treatments per patient, we find 19 strictures among 1950 ablation treatments, or an estimate of 1 stricture per 100 ablation treatments. In the most rigorously conducted study, by Shaheen and colleagues,[9] strictures occurred in 6.4% of patients, or 1 stricture per 55 ablations. Even in accepting the higher estimate, RFA still compares favorably with PDT, in which the rate of strictures has been reported to be as high as 36%.[10,32] In cryotherapy, the rate of strictures has ranged from 3% to 10% of patients in case series, which is comparable with RFA.[26,33] However, further controlled studies are necessary to adequately determine the safety profile of cryotherapy. Nevertheless, RFA is not rec-ommended in patients whose anatomy limits the ability to make adequate tissue contact with the probe, such as with significant strictures. Thus, there may be a role for ablation with cryotherapy in patients not suitable for RFA therapy.

A major concern for ablative procedures is that incompletely ablated Barrett epithelium could have residual metaplastic tissue buried under the squamous neoepithelium. These concerns are fueled by case reports of dysplasia and adenocarcinoma in subsquamous metaplastic glands.[34,35] The clinical implications of subsquamous metaplasia are unknown. Recent studies have shown a low risk of malignant transformation, and generally higher-grade dysplasia can be found in other biopsies from the esophagus that are not buried.[36,37] RFA has shown a low rate of postablation subsquamous metaplasia, as well as an ability to eradicate preablation subsquamous metaplasia. In the AIM Dysplasia trial, 25.2% of patients had buried metaplasia before any intervention.[9] At 12 months, it became less prevalent among those receiving ablation (5.1%) and more prevalent among those receiving the sham procedure (40.0%). Twelve of 14 studies reporting on subsquamous metaplasia found zero cases after ablation, which raises concern for false negatives caused by faulty sampling. However, reassurance is given by a study in which a combination of primary and keyhole biopsies, as well as endoscopic resection, were used to assess for subsquamous metaplasia after RFA.[38] Despite having biopsy specimens that reached the lamina propria among more than 37% of 194 primary biopsies, 51% of 177 keyhole biopsies, and 100% of endoscopic resections, there were zero cases of subsquamous metaplasia identified after RFA. By comparison, patients undergoing PDT have been reported to have a rate of buried metaplasia exceeding 30%.[37,39] The rate of subsquamous metaplasia following cryotherapy has not yet been adequately assessed in clinical trials.

Similar to subsquamous metaplasia, there is concern for the possibility of dysplasia or cancer of the gastric cardia following ablation, which has been reported in patients undergoing thermal ablation.[40,41] Data on this risk are scant; the randomized controlled trial reported a single cardia cancer in a patient undergoing RFA, which was resected for cure with EMR.[9] None of the clinical trials have specifically reported on biopsies taken from the cardia, and thus further information is needed to determine the degree to which this entity occurs following RFA.

Regarding the risk of bleeding after RFA, among 14 studies that reported data on this outcome, there were 12 total cases of bleeding described. Among 930 patients, the rate was 1.3%. Excluding the 2 studies that did not report the number of ablation treatments per patient, there were 11 cases among 1725 ablations, or approximately 1 case per 150 ablations. Most cases of bleeding occurred in the setting of concurrent antiplatelet therapy that could not be discontinued for the procedure, because of the strength of its indication (such as severe coronary artery disease). Among the 12 cases of reported bleeding, 2 required endoscopic intervention and 1 required overnight hospitalization for observation. Otherwise, all reports of bleeding were self-limited, did not require blood transfusion, and the patients were discharged the same day.

Overall, patients tolerated the procedure well. As detailed in **Table 2**, among studies reporting on patient tolerability, 8.9% reported chest pain or dysphagia, and 7.5% reported nausea. However, varying thresholds of reporting adverse events between the studies make these numbers difficult to interpret. For example, in the study by Shaheen and colleagues,[9] 2 cases of severe chest pain were reported. Both of these cases required overnight hospitalization for evaluation. By contrast, Sharma and colleagues[30] reported all incident complaints of chest pain or dysphagia. Likely more telling is that discomfort scores, which were solicited from the patients after ablation, generally returned to zero between post-ablation day 4 and 8.[9,11,30] In the study by Sharma and colleagues,[30] acetaminophen was used for discomfort by 44% on day 1 and 6% on day 7.

ENDOSCOPIC RESECTION AND RFA

Endoscopic resection (ER) of BE is an alternative modality that may be used in lieu of, or in combination with, RFA for mucosal ablation. In addition to treating BE, ER has the advantage of providing diagnostic specimens for review by a pathologist, allowing more accurate staging of disease. However, focal ER alone of nodular HGD or early cancer leaves residual BE that remains at risk for cancer.[42] As a result, complete eradication of all BE is the preferred approach, as shown by the significantly lower rates of metachronous neoplasia in a study by Pech and colleagues.[43]

In the treatment of BE, complete resection of all evident BE by ER, known as step-wise radical endoscopic resection (SRER), and focal ER combined with RFA are competing alternatives for complete eradication. Both have shown efficacy on par with isolated RFA.[17,44] The challenge to both modalities has been in complication rates. In a recent multicenter randomized trial comparing SRER with RFA plus focal ER, SRER had an unacceptably high rate of bleeding (23%) and symptomatic esophageal stenosis (86%).[45] In that same trial, RFA with focal ER had a 14% rate of esophageal stenosis, higher than the 2.2% aggregate rate that we report for isolated RFA, but much lower than that reported for SRER. However, other studies of RFA with focal ER have yielded lower rates of esophageal stenosis.[17] Therefore, for complete eradication of BE, RFA has shown comparable efficacy with a superior side effect profile compared with SRER.

In the treatment of nodular Barrett mucosa, RFA is less attractive as first-line therapy because of the superficial nature of the tissue injury and the inability to ensure that all neoplastic tissue is treated. Therefore, focal ER is a necessary first step to remove nodularity. Although not studied with regard to RFA, Pech and colleagues[43] showed that focal ER with subsequent esophageal ablation was associated with significantly lower disease recurrence (16.5%) than rates in subjects without subsequent ablation (29.9%). Given these data, it is reasonable that all patients with nodular BE receive ablative therapy following focal ER of nodular dysplastic BE.

SUMMARY

Studies in the last several years have consistently shown RFA to be effective, safe, and well tolerated in the treatment of nondysplastic and dysplastic BE. The results found at academic medical centers have been reproduced in the community setting.[15] RFA provides a safe and cost-effective alternative to surgery or surveillance in the management of HGD. Its role in the setting of low-grade and nondysplastic disease is less clear, but there is evidence of durable reversion and cost-effectiveness in these groups. Presumably, the value of ablative therapy in LGD is greater than that in nondysplastic disease, at least to the degree to which cancer risk is higher in LGD than in nondysplastic disease. Until further data are available in subjects with less advanced disease, decision making will likely be on a case-by-case basis, considering multiple patient factors, such as age, extent of disease, and psychological factors, and must acknowledge our lack of information regarding the effect of the therapy on cancer prevention.

Further studies should be performed to determine the durability of RFA and the appropriate surveillance protocol following ablation. Prospective clinical trials of cryoablation are warranted, and, if they substantiate effectiveness, possibly a head-to-head study with RFA to more adequately develop the role of each in the management of BE. Ideally, a study comparing ablation with surgery, with the primary endpoint being mortality, would be helpful to definitively clarify the role of each, although such a trial may be difficult to execute if patients are unwilling to randomize. Regarding BE, future study should focus on developing better predictive models for disease progression as well as clarifying the clinical implications of subsquamous metaplasia and whether gastric cardia biopsies should be routinely obtained following ablation. Societal guidelines should be updated to reflect the developing evidence supporting ablation.

Based on the available data and knowledge of RFA versus competing treatment strategies, RFA should be given serious consideration as first-line therapy for patients with HGD. In patients with LGD, substantial evidence supports RFA, including a good safety profile and high reversion rates, but no data on a cancer preventative effect are available. Therefore, treatment in the setting of LGD requires a shared decision-making model, acknowledging what is not known. In NDBE, the risk of cancer is even lower and, again, there are no data regarding cancer prevention. A broad recommendation for ablation in the setting of nondysplastic disease cannot presently be made, but it may be appropriate for selected patients, especially if further efforts at risk stratification identify a higher-risk subset within this group.

ACKNOWLEDGMENTS

This research was supported, in part, by the National Institutes of Health (T32 DK07634).

REFERENCES

1. Ronkainen J, Aro P, Storskrubb T, et al. Prevalence of Barrett's esophagus in the general population: an endoscopic study. Gastroenterology 2005;129(6): 1825–31.
2. Pohl H, Welch HG. The role of overdiagnosis and reclassification in the marked increase of esophageal adenocarcinoma incidence. J Natl Cancer Inst 2005; 97(2):142–6.
3. Eloubeidi MA, Mason AC, Desmond RA, et al. Temporal trends (1973–1997) in survival of patients with esophageal adenocarcinoma in the United States: a glimmer of hope? Am J Gastroenterol 2003;98(7):1627–33.
4. Williams VA, Watson TJ, Herbella FA, et al. Esophagectomy for high grade dysplasia is safe, curative, and results in good alimentary outcome. J Gastrointest Surg 2007;11(12):1589–97.
5. Schnell TG, Sontag SJ, Chejfec G, et al. Long-term nonsurgical management of Barrett's esophagus with high-grade dysplasia. Gastroenterology 2001;120(7): 1607–19.
6. Brandt LJ, Kauvar DR. Laser-induced transient regression of Barrett's epithelium. Gastrointest Endosc 1992;38(5):619–22.
7. Berenson MM, Johnson TD, Markowitz NR, et al. Restoration of squamous mucosa after ablation of Barrett's esophageal epithelium. Gastroenterology 1993;104(6):1686–91.
8. Rice TW, Falk GW, Achkar E, et al. Surgical management of high-grade dysplasia in Barrett's esophagus. Am J Gastroenterol 1993;88(11):1832–6.
9. Shaheen NJ, Sharma P, Overholt BF, et al. Radiofrequency ablation in Barrett's esophagus with dysplasia. N Engl J Med 2009;360(22):2277–88.
10. Overholt BF, Lightdale CJ, Wang KK, et al. Photodynamic therapy with porfimer sodium for ablation of high-grade dysplasia in Barrett's esophagus: international, partially blinded, randomized phase III trial. Gastrointest Endosc 2005;62(4): 488–98.

11. Fleischer DE, Overholt BF, Sharma VK, et al. Endoscopic ablation of Barrett's esophagus: a multicenter study with 2.5-year follow-up. Gastrointest Endosc 2008;68(5):867–76.

12. Goldberg SN. Radiofrequency tumor ablation: principles and techniques. Eur J Ultrasound 2001;13(2):129–47.

13. Nath S, Haines DE. Biophysics and pathology of catheter energy delivery systems. Prog Cardiovasc Dis 1995;37(4):185–204.

14. Dunkin BJ, Martinez J, Bejarano PA, et al. Thin-layer ablation of human esophageal epithelium using a bipolar radiofrequency balloon device. Surg Endosc 2006;20(1):125–30.

15. Lyday WD, Corbett FS, Kuperman DA, et al. Radiofrequency ablation of Barrett's esophagus: outcomes of 429 patients from a multicenter community practice registry. Endoscopy 2010;42(4):272–8.

16. Vassiliou MC, von Renteln D, Wiener DC, et al. Treatment of ultralong-segment Barrett's using focal and balloon-based radiofrequency ablation. Surg Endosc 2010;24(4):786–91.

17. Pouw RE, Wirths K, Eisendrath P, et al. Efficacy of radiofrequency ablation combined with endoscopic resection for Barrett's esophagus with early neoplasia. Clin Gastroenterol Hepatol 2010;8(1):23–9.

18. Velanovich V. Endoscopic endoluminal radiofrequency ablation of Barrett's esophagus: initial results and lessons learned. Surg Endosc 2009;23(10):2175–80.

19. Ganz RA, Overholt BF, Sharma VK, et al. Circumferential ablation of Barrett's esophagus that contains high-grade dysplasia: a U.S. multicenter registry. Gastrointest Endosc 2008;68(1):35–40.

20. Gondrie JJ, Pouw RE, Sondermeijer CM, et al. Stepwise circumferential and focal ablation of Barrett's esophagus with high-grade dysplasia: results of the first prospective series of 11 patients. Endoscopy 2008;40(5):359–69.

21. Gondrie JJ, Pouw RE, Sondermeijer CM, et al. Effective treatment of early Barrett's neoplasia with stepwise circumferential and focal ablation using the HALO system. Endoscopy 2008;40(5):370–9.

22. Hernandez JC, Reicher S, Chung D, et al. Pilot series of radiofrequency ablation of Barrett's esophagus with or without neoplasia. Endoscopy 2008;40(5):388–92.

23. Roorda AK, Marcus SN, Triadafilopoulos G. Early experience with radiofrequency energy ablation therapy for Barrett's esophagus with and without dysplasia. Dis Esophagus 2007;20(6):516–22.

24. Sharma VK, Jae Kim H, Das A, et al. Circumferential and focal ablation of Barrett's esophagus containing dysplasia. Am J Gastroenterol 2009;104(2):310–7.

25. Shaheen NJ, Fleischer DE, Eisen GM, et al. Durability of epithelial reversion after radiofrequency ablation: follow-up of the AIM dysplasia trial. Gastroenterology 2010;138(5 Suppl 1):S16–7.

26. Shaheen NJ, Greenwald BD, Peery AF, et al. Safety and efficacy of endoscopic spray cryotherapy for Barrett's esophagus with high-grade dysplasia. Gastrointest Endosc 2010;71(4):680–5.

27. Inadomi JM, Somsouk M, Madanick RD, et al. A cost-utility analysis of ablative therapy for Barrett's esophagus. Gastroenterology 2009;136(7):2101–14, e2101–6.

28. Eldaif SM, Lin E, Singh KA, et al. Radiofrequency ablation of Barrett's esophagus: short-term results. Ann Thorac Surg 2009;87(2):405–10 [discussion: 410–1].

29. Sharma VK, Kim HJ, Das A, et al. A prospective pilot trial of ablation of Barrett's esophagus with low-grade dysplasia using stepwise circumferential and focal ablation (HALO system). Endoscopy 2008;40(5):380–7.

30. Sharma VK, Wang KK, Overholt BF, et al. Balloon-based, circumferential, endoscopic radiofrequency ablation of Barrett's esophagus: 1-year follow-up of 100 patients. Gastrointest Endosc 2007;65(2):185–95.

31. Sharma P, Falk GW, Weston AP, et al. Dysplasia and cancer in a large multicenter cohort of patients with Barrett's esophagus. Clin Gastroenterol Hepatol 2006;4(5): 566–72.

32. Prasad GA, Wang KK, Buttar NS, et al. Predictors of stricture formation after photodynamic therapy for high-grade dysplasia in Barrett's esophagus. Gastrointest Endosc 2007;65(1):60–6.

33. Dumot JA, Vargo JJ 2nd, Falk GW, et al. An open-label, prospective trial of cryospray ablation for Barrett's esophagus high-grade dysplasia and early esophageal cancer in high-risk patients. Gastrointest Endosc 2009;70(4):635–44.

34. Mino-Kenudson M, Ban S, Ohana M, et al. Buried dysplasia and early adenocarcinoma arising in Barrett esophagus after porfimer-photodynamic therapy. Am J Surg Pathol 2007;31(3):403–9.

35. Van Laethem JL, Peny MO, Salmon I, et al. Intramucosal adenocarcinoma arising under squamous re-epithelialisation of Barrett's oesophagus. Gut 2000;46(4): 574–7.

36. Hornick JL, Mino-Kenudson M, Lauwers GY, et al. Buried Barrett's epithelium following photodynamic therapy shows reduced crypt proliferation and absence of DNA content abnormalities. Am J Gastroenterol 2008;103(1):38–47.

37. Bronner MP, Overholt BF, Taylor SL, et al. Squamous overgrowth is not a safety concern for photodynamic therapy for Barrett's esophagus with high-grade dysplasia. Gastroenterology 2009;136(1):56–64 [quiz: 351–2].

38. Pouw RE, Gondrie JJ, Rygiel AM, et al. Properties of the neosquamous epithelium after radiofrequency ablation of Barrett's esophagus containing neoplasia. Am J Gastroenterol 2009;104(6):1366–73.

39. Peters F, Kara M, Rosmolen W, et al. Poor results of 5-aminolevulinic acid-photodynamic therapy for residual high-grade dysplasia and early cancer in Barrett esophagus after endoscopic resection. Endoscopy 2005;37(5):418–24.

40. Sampliner RE, Camargo E, Prasad AR. Association of ablation of Barrett's esophagus with high grade dysplasia and adenocarcinoma of the gastric cardia. Dis Esophagus 2006;19(4):277–9.

41. Weston AP, Sharma P, Banerjee S, et al. Visible endoscopic and histologic changes in the cardia, before and after complete Barrett's esophagus ablation. Gastrointest Endosc 2005;61(4):515–21.

42. May A, Gossner L, Pech O, et al. Local endoscopic therapy for intraepithelial high-grade neoplasia and early adenocarcinoma in Barrett's oesophagus: acute-phase and intermediate results of a new treatment approach. Eur J Gastroenterol Hepatol 2002;14(10):1085–91.

43. Pech O, Behrens A, May A, et al. Long-term results and risk factor analysis for recurrence after curative endoscopic therapy in 349 patients with high-grade intraepithelial neoplasia and mucosal adenocarcinoma in Barrett's oesophagus. Gut 2008;57(9):1200–6.

44. Pouw RE, Seewald S, Gondrie JJ, et al. Stepwise radical endoscopic resection for eradication of Barrett's oesophagus with early neoplasia in a cohort of 169 patients. Gut 2010;59(9):1169–77.

45. Van Vilsteren FG, Pouw RE, Seewald S, et al. A multi-center randomized trial comparing stepwise radical endoscopic resection versus radiofrequency ablation for Barrett esophagus containing high-grade dysplasia and/or early cancer. Gastrointest Endosc 2009;69(5):AB133–4.

Cryotherapy for Barrett's Esophagus: Who, How, and Why?

Ann M. Chen, MD[a], Pankaj J. Pasricha, MD[b],*

KEYWORDS

• Cryotherapy • Cryoablation • Barrett's esophagus

Approximately 16,500 Americans are diagnosed with esophageal cancer and 14,500 die of this malignancy each year.[1] The incidence of esophageal adenocarcinoma has continued to rise dramatically over the past 4 decades and is growing at a rate faster than that of any other cancer in the United States. Barrett's esophagus (BE) is a well-known risk factor in the development of esophageal adenocarcinoma. In the absence of dysplasia, BE is associated with an increased esophageal cancer risk of approximately 0.5% per patient-year. With the presence of high-grade dysplasia (HGD), however, the risk of progression to cancer may be as high as 10% per patient-year.[2] Traditionally, surgery with esophagectomy has been the mainstay of treatment for patients found with HGD; however, many patients are elderly and deemed to be poor surgical candidates. In addition, esophagectomy is associated with significant morbidity and mortality and recent reports have shown recurrence of Barrett metaplasia in as high as 18% of patients after "curative" esophagectomy despite high-dose acid suppressive medications.[3] Therefore, there is increasing interest and research in endoscopic treatments of BE. Cryoablation has long been used to treat a wide variety of dermatologic and gynecologic conditions for more than half a century. Not until recently, however, was the application of cryotherapy in gastroenterology seriously investigated, particularly in the treatment of dysplastic BE and early esophageal cancer. This article focuses on current understanding and results of cryotherapy in the treatment of BE.

Dr Ann Chen has nothing to disclose.
Dr Jay Pasricha is an inventor of Polar Wand cryoablation device (GI Supply, Camp Hill, Pennsylvania) and a consultant for the company.
[a] Division of Gastroenterology and Hepatology, Stanford University School of Medicine, Stanford University Medical Center, 450 Broadway Street, Pavilion C, 4th Floor, MC 6341, Redwood City, CA 94063, USA
[b] Division of Gastroenterology and Hepatology, Stanford University School of Medicine, Stanford University Medical Center, Alway Building, Room M211, 300 Pasteur Drive, MC 5187, Stanford, CA 94305, USA
* Corresponding author.
E-mail address: pasricha@stanford.edu

Gastrointest Endoscopy Clin N Am 21 (2011) 111–118
doi:10.1016/j.giec.2010.09.007
1052-5157/11/$ – see front matter © 2011 Elsevier Inc. All rights reserved.

giendo.theclinics.com

PRINCIPLES AND MECHANISMS OF CRYOTHERAPY ABLATION

Cryotherapy is the application of exceptionally cold temperatures to destroy targeted tissue. Tissue destruction from repeated cycles of rapid freezing followed by slow thawing occurs on a cellular and molecular level. At temperatures between −76°C and −158°C, cryotherapy can induce cellular apoptosis.[4] The exact mechanism and biology underlying tissue injury is complex and incompletely understood. As the temperature drops to the freezing point, water in the extracellular matrix forms ice crystals and creates a hypertonic environment causing water to leave the cells by osmosis. Intracellular dehydration and shrinkage ensue. With further freezing, intracellular ice crystallization also occurs, leading to protein denaturation and shearing of the organelles and cytoskeleton.[5] During the thawing process, a brief period of extracellular hypotonicity results in a reverse osmotic gradient, which causes water to rush into the cells rapidly leading to cellular swelling and eventual rupture of the cell membrane. Effects of cryotherapy on cellular injury are dependent on several factors, including the rate of cooling and thawing, the lowest tissue temperature achieved, the water content of the cells, and the number of freeze-thaw cycles.[6] The drop in tissue temperature occurs more quickly with each freeze-thaw cycle and leads to increased depth and volume of the area affected.

Delayed injurious effects of cryotherapy are as important in tissue destruction as the immediate effects and occur hours to days after treatment. Freezing causes vasoconstriction and modification of vascular endothelium, resulting in a cascade of events including increased vascular wall permeability, decreased blood flow, platelet aggregation, and formation of microthrombi. With the loss of microcirculation, a wide area of progressive cellular anoxia and hemorrhagic necrosis results in apoptosis of even cells that may have survived the initial freezing.[7] Furthermore, immune-related processes also may contribute to the success of delayed effects of cryotherapy on malignant tumors. Cancer cells outside of the ablation area have been shown to undergo apoptosis by cryotherapy-induced antitumor response.[8,9] It has been proposed that cryoimmunity may be achieved via increases in tumor antigens against a backdrop of a significant inflammatory microenvironment created during the cryoablative process, which then results in cytotoxic T-cell proliferation and enhanced Th1 response.[10] Although cryoimmunity has not been specifically studied in gastrointestinal cancers, the possibility of enhanced antitumor immunogenicity makes cryotherapy particularly attractive compared with other endoscopic ablation therapies.

ENDOSCOPIC CRYOTHERAPY DEVICES

The major technical advantage of cryotherapy in comparison with other ablative technologies is the ability to spray the mucosa at will, producing rapid injury of fairly large areas *without* the need for contact. In contrast, the success of most thermal ablation techniques is dependent on precise close contact between the ablation probe and esophageal mucosa. Although studies are needed, cryotherapy in theory may be the preferred modality to treat lesions in the gastroesophageal junction and in patients with a slightly tortuous esophageal anatomy where precise physical contact between the surface of the ablation probe and the mucosa is very difficult to maintain. The major disadvantage of cryotherapy compared with thermal ablation is the large volume of cryogen gas exiting the catheter, which increases risks of perforation unless adequate venting is established. Pasricha and colleagues[11] first described a through-the-scope probe-based cryotherapeutic device (Cryomedical Sciences Inc, Bethesda, MD, USA) consisting of a long, insulated catheter through which liquid nitrogen is delivered near its saturation temperature of $-196°C$. Clinical application of the initial prototype was limited because of restricted catheter maneuverability caused by excessive endoscopic rigidity from delivery of liquid nitrogen at very low temperature. The investigators then went on to describe a second prototype that used cryogenic refrigerant at or near ambient temperature, based on the Joule Thomson effect, whereby high-pressured gas, in this case carbon dioxide (CO_2), is forced at or near ambient temperature through the catheter and upon reaching the distal tip, a sudden and rapid expansion of the gas from a higher pressure to atmospheric pressure causes a massive drop in temperature. More recently, this invention was incorporated into the Polar Wand cryotherapy device (GI Supply, Camp Hill, PA, USA) using CO_2 gas as a cooling agent (**Fig. 1**). At flow conditions of 6 to 8 L/min, end effector temperatures of $-78°C$ can be achieved. The ablation catheter is passed though the working channel and a suction catheter is attached to the tip of the endo-scope for decompression. In contrast to a liquid nitrogen–based cryoablation system (see the following paragraph), the cryocatheter in the accessory channel remains at ambient temperature, thus preserving normal endoscopic maneuver-ability. Furthermore, expensive cryogen holding tanks used to contain liquid nitrogen are not necessary when using a CO_2-based system.

The CryoSpray Ablation System (CSA Medical, Inc, Baltimore, MD, USA) is an alternative method to deliver cryotherapy and consists of a 7F catheter manufac-tured from a special polymer (**Fig. 2**). With this system, a dual-lumen orogastric suction tube is inserted into the stomach for active suction and passive luminal decompression. Multiple distal ports and side holes along the cryo decompression tube allow for both gastric and esophageal decompression. Luminal decompres-sion is imperative to prevent perforation because liquid nitrogen can expand into 6 to 8 L of gas during each 20 seconds of treatment. The endoscopist controls the cryoablation and suction decompression with a foot pedal provided with the system.

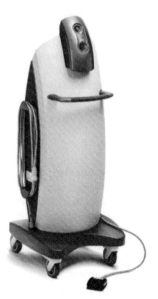

Fig. 1. Polar Wand CO_2-based cryotherapy system. (*Courtesy of* GI Supply, Camp Hill, PA; with permission.)

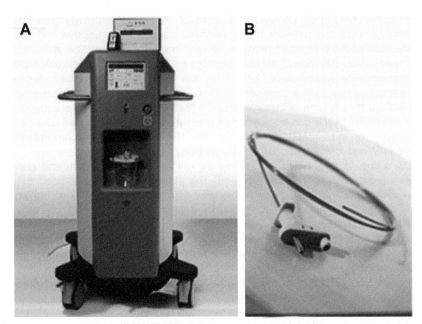

Fig. 2. CryoSpray liquid nitrogen ablation system. The console (*A*) and catheter (*B*) are shown. The catheter is available in either straight or directional tip. (*Courtesy of* CSA Medical, Baltimore, MD, Inc; with permission.)

DOSIMETRY

Initial CO_2 dosimetry experiments using 8 pigs showed that after 15 seconds of cryoablation, esophageal necrosis was limited to the mucosa.[12] The depth of injury was extended into the submucosa if the duration of treatment was increased to 15 to 30 seconds. Treatment for 45 to 60 seconds results in necrosis into the muscularis propria and frank transmural necrosis occurred after 120 seconds of application. In addition to the duration of ablation, the number of freeze-thaw cycles also affects the depth and extent of injury. In a study using liquid nitrogen cryoablation of the pig esophagus, treatment for 20 seconds each over 2 cycles produced a mean depth of injury of 5.3 mm, whereas treatment for 10 seconds each over 4 cycles resulted in a mean depth of injury of 4.75 mm.[13]

TECHNIQUE AND COMPLICATIONS

Cryoablation can be performed using standard conscious sedation but monitored anesthesia care may be considered for patients with a long segment of dysplastic Barrett's esophagus. In general, 5 to 6 cm of the esophagus may be treated in 45 to 60 minutes. Anticoagulation and nonsteroidal anti-inflammatory medications should be stopped for 1 week before the procedure. Ideally, 48-hour pH manometry on proton pump inhibitors should be performed before ablation and if acid breakthrough is found, medications adjusted to ensure adequate acid suppression for optimal mucosal healing after cryotherapy treatment.

For procedures involving CryoSpray, the decompression catheter is placed into the stomach over a guide wire after routine endoscopic examination. The ablation catheter is then inserted through the accessory channel of the endoscope and activated by stepping on the foot pedal. Suction is also initiated at the time of cryoablation with the foot pedal and the black line on the suction tube should be positioned at the gastroesophageal junction for optimal decompression. Esophageal peristaltic contractions and frost caused by the liquid nitrogen gas may obscure endoscopic visualization; therefore, a soft clear cap (Olympus America, Center Valley, PA, USA) is sometimes placed at the tip of the endoscope to lessen these problems. Each cycle of cryogen spray is applied continuously to a 2 × 2-cm area for approximately 15 to 20 seconds, then allowed to completely thaw for 5 seconds or so before the cycle is repeated again in the same area 3 to 4 times. It is ideal to achieve mucosal ice crystal formation during the freeze cycle and punctuate erythema during the thaw cycle (**Fig. 3**). Slight overlapping of 2 treatment areas has not been shown to be a significant problem and treatment may be repeated every 6 to 8 weeks until adequate results are achieved. At the end of each treatment session, the catheter is warmed with the heat cycle provided with the system before removal from the endoscope.

The technique for Polar Wand cryotherapy is similar to CryoSpray except, as previously mentioned, the suction catheter is attached to the tip of the endoscope and thus obviates the problem of treatment areas obstructed by the decompression tube. The endoscope along with the attached decompression catheter is then advanced into the stomach for decompression after each freezing cycle. In contrast to liquid nitrogen–based systems, the cryocatheter does not need warming before removal from the endoscope. No standard dosimetry has been established for the CO_2 system but ablation for 15 seconds times 8 cycles has been proposed based on preliminary animal studies in mice (Mimi Canto, MD, Baltimore, MD, personal communication, May 2010).

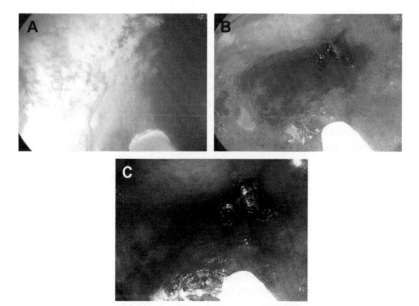

Fig. 3. Endoscopic images of cryotherapy for Barrett's esophagus with CO_2-based system. (*A*) Ice crystal formation is visible on the surface of the mucosa during the freeze cycle. (*B*) Immediately after thawing, reactive mucosal hyperemia owing to transient ischemic injury is seen endoscopically. (*C*) Narrow band imaging technology can be used to enhance visualization of postablation hyperemia.

Contraindications to esophageal cryotherapy ablation include mucosal breaks, coagulopathy, chronic anticoagulation, and other contraindications to standard upper endoscopy. Cryoablation in the setting of pregnancy has not been well studied and should therefore not be performed. When retained gastric contents are found, the procedure should be rescheduled, as food particles may cause blockage of the suction tube and prevent adequate decompression. Increased risks of perforation may also occur in patients with restricted volume or decreased distensibility of the gastrointestinal tract; therefore, patients with conditions such as post–gastric bypass surgical anatomy and eosinophilic esophagitis should not undergo cryoablation therapy.

Complications after cryoablation are generally mild and self-limited. Chest pain and dysphagia may occur in up to 50% of patients, especially in those with a long segment of Barrett's esophagus treated. Viscous lidocaine and hydrocodone may be given but are rarely needed. Perforations and esophageal strictures have been reported but occur in fewer than 5% of patients.

CLINICAL RESULTS TO DATE

In a pilot study reported by Johnston and colleagues,[14] liquid nitrogen–based cryotherapy was evaluated for its safety and efficacy in 11 patients with varying lengths of BE (mean 4.6 cm, range 1–8 cm) and degrees of dysplasia (none to mulitfocal high-grade). Cryotherapy was applied hemicircumferentially to the distal esophagus with 2 repeat freezing applications of 20 seconds each. Treatment was repeated monthly until reversal (at least 1 cm length reduction) or complete reversal (no endoscopic evidence of BE) was confirmed by biopsy. The mean number of cryotherapy treatments was 3.6 (range 1–6). In this series, 9 of 11 patients completed the protocol and 78% (7 of 9) of them achieved complete histologic resolution of BE at 6-month follow-up. Complications were mild, including 2 patients with self-limited esophageal ulcers and 2 others with 1 day of chest discomfort and mild dysphagia.

In a more recent study,[15] liquid nitrogen CryoSpray was also evaluated in the treatment of BE with HGD and early intramucosal carcinoma (IMCA). Endoscopic mucosal resection was performed to eradicate nodular areas before ablation. At median follow-up of 12 months, 27 (90%) of 30 patients had downgrading of histology. This response was seen in 92% of HGD patients and 80% of IMCA patients. Complete resolution of dysplasia was seen in 32% of HGD patients and 40% of IMCA patients. The most common complication from treatment was chest pain, which was reported in 7 (25%) patients, 3 of whom required a short course of narcotic analgesics. There were also 3 patients who developed mild strictures requiring endoscopic dilation. Gastric perforation occurred in a patient with Marfan syndrome caused by overdistension of the stomach who recovered after laparotomy. This complication occurred early in the study with a prototype device and single-lumen gastric decompression tube. Overall 97.3% (36 of 37) treated resumed normal activity and diet the next day.

Similar success has been reported with CO_2 cryotherapy. Canto and colleagues[16] treated 44 patients with HGD or IMCA who were deemed nonsurgical candidates. Twenty-five of these patients had failed prior endoscopic treatment with radiofrequency, mucosal resection, or photodynamic therapy. The mean length of BE was 4.8 cm and a mean of 6 treatment sessions (range 1–10) were performed. For those who completed cryotherapy treatment, complete resolution was seen in (22/23) 95.6% in BE, (22/23) 95.6% in LGD, and (21/23) 91.3% in HGD. Only 2 patients in this study reported mild transient chest discomfort and no serious adverse events were noted.

A large retrospective study at 9 centers of 98 patients who underwent 333 treatments for BE with HGD using liquid nitrogen CryoSpray showed high efficacy and low complication rate.[17] In this study, 14% of the patients had failed prior ablation therapies. There were 2 patients who developed chest pain requiring oral narcotics and 3 patients with esophageal strictures requiring dilation. One subject was hospitalized for self-limited bright red blood per rectum and no esophageal perforations were reported. Sixty subjects had completed cryotherapy treatments of which 58 (97%) had complete eradication of HGD, 52 (87%) had complete eradication of all dysplasia, and 34 (57%) had complete eradication of all intestinal metaplasia. Subsquamous BE was found in 2 subjects (3%).

Last, there is increasing support also for the use of cryotherapy in nonresectable esophageal adenocarcinoma. A retrospective study of 79 nonsurgical, cancer patients (T1-60, T2-16, T3/T4-3) at 10 centers was recently reported for liquid nitrogen CryoSpray.[18] For the 49 patients completing therapy, a local cancer eradication rate of 61.2% and 75.0% for mucosal cancers was achieved with an average of 3 treatment sessions. Tumor burden averaged 4 cm, and prior therapy had failed in 67% of these subjects. No serious adverse events were reported. Benign stricture developed in 10 (13%), with prior esophageal narrowing from previous endoscopic resection, radiotherapy, or photodynamic therapy noted in 9 of 10 subjects.

SUMMARY

Cryotherapy ablation is a new and exciting minimally invasive approach to endoscopic treatment of dysplastic BE. The mechanism of inducing cellular apoptosis and ischemic injury is unique compared with other ablative technologies. In addition, the relatively low cost, ease of use, high efficacy, and low complication rates make cryotherapy a particularly attractive therapy of choice. Further studies on optimal dosimetry and larger as well as long-term clinical trials are under way. Finally, ablation, including cryothearpy in nondysplastic BE is controversial because of low risks of disease progression to malignancy. However, an excellent safety and efficacy profile may justify treatment of nondysplastic Barrett's esophagus, which, after all, is precursor to a serious malignant disease rather than waiting for it to progress. From a cost-effective standpoint, eradication rather than surveillance may also be the preferred course if complete removal of intestinal metaplasia is maintained over time. Randomized controlled trials as wells as biomarkers that predict lesions at high risk of progression are desperately needed to help answer some very important questions in the management of a potentially life-threatening disease with rapidly rising incidence.

REFERENCES

1. American Cancer Society. Cancer facts and figures 2009. Atlanta (GA): American Cancer Society; 2009.
2. Shaheen NJ, Richter JE. Barrett's oesophagus. Lancet 2009;373:850–61.
3. Wolfsen HC, Hemminger LL, DeVault KR. Recurrent Barrett's esophagus and adenocarcinoma after esophagectomy. BMC Gastroenterol 2004;4:18.
4. Gage AA, Baust J. Mechanisms of tissue injury in cryosurgery. Cryobiology 1998; 37(3):171–86.
5. Rubinsky B. The freezing process and mechanism of tissue damage. In: Onik GM, Rubinsky B, Watson F, Albin RJ, editors. Quality percutaneous prostate cryoablation. St. Louis (MO): Medical Publishing; 1995. p. 49.
6. Mazur P. Cryobiology: the freezing of biological systems. Science 1970;168(934): 939–49.

7. Whittaker DK. Mechanism of tissue destruction following cryosurgery. Ann R Coll Surg Engl 1984;66(5):313–8.

8. Ablin RJ, Soanes WA, Gonder MJ. Elution of in vivo bound antiprostatic epithelial antibodies following multiple cryotherapy of carcinoma of prostate. Urology 1973; 2:276–9.

9. Hollister WR, Mathew AJ, Baust JG, et al. Effects of freezing on cell viability and mechanism of cell death in a human prostate cell line. Mol Urol 1998;2(1):3–18.

10. Machlenkin A, Goldberger O, Tirosh B, et al. Combined dendritic cell cryotherapy of tumor induces systemic antimetastatic immunity. Clin Cancer Res 2005;11(13): 4955–61.

11. Pasricha PJ, Hill S, Wadwa KS, et al. Endoscopic cryotherapy: experimental results and first clinical use. Gastrointest Endosc 1999;49(5):627–31.

12. Raju GS, Ahmed I, Xiao SY, et al. Graded esophageal mucosal ablation with cryotherapy, and the protective effects of submucosal saline. Endoscopy 2005;37(6): 523–6.

13. Johnston L, Johnston MH. Cryospray ablation (CSA) in the esophagus: optimization of dosimetry [abstract]. Am J Gastroenterol 2006;101:S532.

14. Johnston MH, Eastone JA, Horwhat JD, et al. Cryoablation of Barrett's esophagus: a pilot study. Gastrointest Endosc 2005;62(6):842–8.

15. Dumot JA, Vargo JJ, Falk GW, et al. An open-label, prospective trial of cryospray ablation for Barrett's esophagus high-grade dysplasia and early esophageal cancer in high-risk patients. Gastrointest Endosc 2009;70(4):635–44.

16. Canto MI, Gorospe EC, Shin EJ, et al. Carbon dioxide (CO2) Cryotherapy is a safe and effective treatment of Barrett's esophagus (BE) with HGD/intramucosal carcinoma. Gastrointest Endosc 2009;69(5):AB341.

17. Shaheen NJ, Greenwald BD, Peery AF, et al. Safety and efficacy of endoscopic spray cryotherapy for Barrett's esophagus with high-grade dysplasia. Gastrointest Endosc 2010;71(4):680–5.

18. Greenwald BD, Dumot JA, Abrams JA, et al. Endoscopic spray cryotherapy for esophageal cancer: safety and efficacy. Gastrointest Endosc 2010;71(4):686–93.

Endotherapy for Barrett's Esophagus: Which, How, When, and Who?

Jennifer Chennat, MD, Vani J.A. Konda, MD, Irving Waxman, MD*

KEYWORDS

- Barrett's esophagus • Barrett's neoplasia treatment
- Endoscopic mucosal resection
- Endoscopic submucosal dissection • Endoscopic ablation
- Photodynamic therapy • Cyrotherapy
- Radiofrequency ablation

The annual incidence of adenocarcinoma arising in the setting of Barrett's esophagus (BE) is approximately 0.5%.[1–3] Adenocarcinoma related to BE develops by a process of gradual transformation from metaplasia to dysplasia to cancer.[4] The identification of BE in stages of intestinal metaplasia (IM), low-grade dysplasia (LGD), high-grade dysplasia (HGD), intramucosal carcinoma (IMC), and invasive adenocarcinoma is clinically challenging and important because it has profound treatment implications based on the dramatically different prognostic profiles between early neoplasia and more advanced stages. Patients who demonstrate symptoms from adenocarcinoma usually harbor locally advanced disease with an approximate 5-year survival rate of 20%.[5,6]

Because of the suspected risk of harboring occult invasive cancer, esophagectomy has been traditionally recommended as the gold standard treatment for BE with HGD, with previous estimations of occult invasive cancer as high as 40%.[7,8] However, the authors' center previously conducted an analysis that applied strict definitions and standardized criteria of the published literature of patients undergoing prophylactic esophagectomy for the management of HGD. In this analysis, the prevalence of occult submucosal invasive carcinoma in the setting of HGD was 12%, which was much lower than the pooled reported rates of 40%.[9] Previously, because of the lack of effective endoscopic alternatives, esophagectomy was also routinely performed for BE

The authors have nothing to disclose.

Center for Endoscopic Research and Therapeutics (CERT), Section of Gastroenterology, Department of Medicine, The University of Chicago Medical Center, 5758 South Maryland Avenue, MC 9028, Chicago, IL 60637-1463, USA

* Corresponding author. Section of Gastroenterology, Department of Medicine, The University of Chicago Medical Center, 5758 South Maryland Avenue, MC 9028, Chicago, IL 60637–1463.

E-mail address: iwaxman@medicine.bsd.uchicago.edu

giendo.theclinics.com

with IMC, despite a low incidence of lymph node metastasis of less than 1%.[10] However, esophagectomy is associated with significant morbidity and mortality even in high-volume centers.[11,12]

With the advent of endoscopic mucosal resection (EMR) and endoscopic ablative therapies, endoscopic therapy at centers with expertise is now an established treatment of BE-related neoplasia including HGD and IMC. However, when considering endoscopic treatment options, it is critical to distinguish the presence of BE with HGD, IMC, or submucosal invasion. This differentiation of histopathologic status is paramount to appropriate selection of endoscopic therapy choice or further consideration for esophagectomy. Intramucosal cancer is limited to the mucosal lining of the esophageal wall, has only a minimal nodal metastasis risk,[13–16] and may be locally treatable with endoscopic means. The presence of cancer with invasion into the submucosa carries a higher nodal metastasis risk and requires surgery or systemic therapy.[15–18] Therefore, esophagectomy is now reserved for more selected cases with submucosal invasion, evidence of lymph node metastasis, or unsuccessful endoscopic therapy.

With these issues in mind, endoscopic therapies have entered the clinical forefront as acceptable nonsurgical alternatives for HGD and IMC, changing the clinical paradigm of BE early neoplasia management (**Table 1**). Endoscopic therapy for HGD or IMC is performed with the goal of ablating all BE epithelium (both dysplastic and nondysplastic) because of risk of synchronous or metachronous lesion development in the remaining at-risk BE segment.[10] The low risk of cancer for patients with nondysplastic BE or with LGD combined with the risk of possible complications that are associated with endoscopic therapy suggests that ablative therapies do not provide the same level of benefit in this group of patients compared with patients with HGD.[19]

ENDOSCOPIC THERAPEUTIC MODALITIES

Endoscopic therapies can be subdivided into tissue-acquiring and non–tissue acquiring modalities (**Table 2**). Tissue acquisition can be achieved through endoscopic resection, whereas photodynamic therapy (PDT), radiofrequency ablation (RFA), and cryotherapy all ablate tissue without the benefit of histologic specimen retrieval. This article covers a brief technical review of each modality with presentation of pertinent available efficacy and safety data in treating various stages of BE neoplasia. Argon plasma coagulation, multipolar electrocoagulation, and laser therapies are not discussed here because they no longer represent current mainstay therapies, as a result of high BE relapse rates, infrequent usage, or significant risk of buried BE gland development.[20]

Endoscopic Resection

EMR can be performed through a variety of techniques: free-hand, lift-and-cut, cap-assisted, and band-assisted. Injection of saline with a sclerotherapy needle is performed to create a submucosal fluid cushion, and a snare is used to directly entrap the mucosal tissue in the free-hand method. In the lift-and-cut approach, a dual-channel endoscope is used to simultaneously introduce a grasping forceps and snare for lifting and resection. The cap technique involves attaching a clear distal cylindrical device to the tip of the endoscope; this cap has an inner rim in which a crescent-shaped snare is carefully fitted. The target area is injected for submucosal lift, then suction is applied, and tissue is entrapped in the cap by the snare for subsequent mucosal excision. Modifications of the variceal band ligation device embody the band-assisted techniques that allow for injection and then deployment of bands for mucosal pseudopolyp creation. A snare is then introduced and the mucosa is resected either above or below the band.[21]

Table 1
Endoscopic therapies for Barrett's esophagus early neoplasia

	Non–Tissue Acquiring Modalities			Tissue-Acquiring Modalities	
	PDT	RFA	Cryo	EMR	ESD
Indication	HGD	HGD	HGD	HGD/IMC	IMC/?SMC
Technique difficulty	Moderate	Easier	Easier	Difficult	Very difficult
Availability	**	****	**	**	*
Cost	***	****	***	**	*
Strengths	Lower chance of perforation	Ease of use, lower chance of perforation and stricture formation	Ease of use, lower chance of perforation	Tissue acquisition	Tissue acquisition
Limitations	Non–tissue acquiring, availability of photosensitizing agents, sunlight sensitivity, and stricture formation	Non–tissue acquiring, chest pain after procedure	Non–tissue acquiring, nonuniform spray application, risk of gastric/enteral perforation caused by gas insufflation	Higher chance of perforation and bleeding, esophageal stricture formation	Highest chance for perforation, lack of technique education and available endoscopic devices in the United States

* low.
** moderate.
*** high.
**** very high.

Table 2
Current treatments for various stages Barrett's esophagus early neoplasia

	Nondysplastic Barrett's	Low-Grade Dysplasia	High-Grade Dysplasia	Intramucosal Carcinoma	Submucosal Carcinoma
Esophagectomy					Current standard
ESD/ESD		Focal: any visible lesion for staging	Focal: any visible lesion for staging complete	Current standard	Low-risk Sm1 lesions in protocol setting
Ablative Therapies	Protocol setting	Case dependent	Flat mucosa only		

Focal EMR can be performed for endoscopically visible lesions that are suspicious for malignancy. However, several previously published studies on focal resection demonstrated a high rate of synchronous and recurrent lesion development, which ranged from 14% to 47% and increased with longer observation times.[22–29] Because of limited efficacy of focal EMR, complete Barrett's eradication EMR has been advocated and performed in select centers, with the intention of curatively removing all BE epithelium to potentially reduce the risk of synchronous or metachronous lesion development. Complete responses have ranged from 76% to 100%. The complication profile of EMR includes stricture formation incidence rate that approaches 50%, bleeding, and, rarely, perforation. Of note, most esophageal stenoses and bleeding are amenable to endoscopic treatment.[30–33]

The effect of EMR on final histopathologic staging has been highlighted in the authors' center's long-term results with complete Barrett's eradication EMR that revealed initial EMR upstaged 7 (14%) of 49 and downstaged 15 (31%) of 49 of patients' final pathology when compared with pre-EMR biopsy HGD results. Moreover, of the upstaged group, four patients had advanced pathology found after index EMR (either submucosal carcinoma or IMC with lymphatic channel invasion). All four of these patients had visible lesions detected on endoscopy.[31] However, these lesions were not described in the referring physicians' endoscopy reports, and these patients had been recommended by their referring physicians to undergo ablative therapy for presumed BE with HGD solely detected on their biopsies. This is the critical point that distinguishes EMR from all other non–tissue acquiring modalities that would have inadvertently attempted ablation of advanced pathology in the setting of presumed BE HGD treatment.

Endoscopic submucosal dissection (ESD) allows for the en bloc dissection of neoplastic lesions. This technique has been used for the removal of superficial gastric cancers in Japan. This may be a suitable modality for lesions at the gastroesophageal junction or cardia. However, it should be approached with caution in the distal esophagus given the potential for reflux-induced submucosal fibrosis.[34] Yoshinaga and colleagues[35] performed ESD at the gastroesophageal junction in 24 patients for adenocarcinoma (15 with BE) and had no recurrence in their follow-up period, which was a mean of 30 months.

For lesions with superficial submucosal invasion into the sm1 layer, endoscopic resection has been studied in a limited fashion. The Wiesbaden group in Germany classified "low-risk" submucosal cancer as demonstrating invasion into the upper third of the submucosa (sm1), absence of infiltration into lymph vessels and veins, histologic grades G1 and G2, and macroscopic types I and II. Their outcomes of endoscopic resection of these low-risk lesions were described as favorable, with a 5-year survival rate of all 21 patients reaching 66%.[36]

To further investigate the controversy of outcomes of esophageal adenocarcinoma with submucosal invasion, Badreddine and colleagues[37] evaluated esophagectomy specimens from patients with esophageal adenocarcinoma and submucosal invasion. Superficial (upper one third, sm1) and deep (middle third, sm2; deepest third, sm3) submucosal invasion were associated with substantial rates of metastatic lymphadenopathy (12.9% and 20.4%, respectively). Their resulting recommendation was that endoscopic treatment of superficial submucosal adenocarcinoma is not advised for patients who are candidates for surgery.

At present, accurate predictors of nodal spread independent of tumor depth are lacking. These parameters are necessary before recommending endoscopic resection with or without concomitant ablation as curative treatment for even superficial submucosal neoplasia.[38] Therefore, the role of ESD in the setting of BE neoplasia remains to be defined, and should only be performed in research protocolized fashion in centers with expertise in endoscopic excisional techniques and management of potential complications. Additionally, esophagectomy should be readily available at these centers to expeditiously treat complications, such as full-thickness perforation resulting from endoscopic resection.

PDT

The goal of PDT is destruction of tissue through a light-sensitizing reaction sequence. A photosensitizer is first administered, which accumulates in esophageal malignant and premalignant tissue before light activation therapy. The most common photosensitizer is porfimer sodium, and this is delivered intravenously 72 hours before the procedure. Available alternatives are oral 5-aminolevulinic acid and intravenous m-tetrahydroxyphenyl chlorine (mTHPC). On exposure to either bare cylinder or balloon-based diffusing light fibers that are placed alongside the target tissue by endoscopic approach, activation of the photosensitizing agent occurs. The resulting molecular excitation reacts with oxygen to facilitate creation of radical oxygen species that cause eventual cell apoptosis.[39]

In a multicenter trial, BE HGD patients were randomized to either receive twice daily oral omeprazole, 20 mg, with or without porfimer sodium PDT administration. At 5 years follow-up time, PDT was significantly more effective than proton pump inhibition alone in elimination of HGD (77% vs 39%; P<.0001). A secondary outcome assessed was prevention of cancer progression that also showed significant difference, with the PDT–proton pump inhibition group demonstrating half the likelihood of developing cancer and longer time to progression to cancer.[40]

Another porfimer PDT study consisted of 103 patients with LGD, HGD, or IMC with a mean follow-up of 50.65 months (range, 2–122 months). Intention-to-treat success rates were 92.9%, 77.5%, and 44.4% for the respective LGD, HGD, and IMC groups. Three patients (4.6%) developed subsquamous adenocarcinoma. Esophageal strictures occurred in 18% with one session of PDT, 50% with two treatments, and 30% in the overall group.[41]

5-Aminolevulinic acid PDT has shown 97% and 100% complete response rates for treatment of BE with HGD and IMC, respectively, in a median follow-up period of 37 months (interquartile range, 23–55). Disease-free survival of HGD patients was 89%, and 68% in patients with IMC. The calculated 5-year survival was 97% for HGD and 80% for IMC, but no deaths were related to Barrett's neoplasia.[42]

In a pilot study of PDT using mTHPC for HGD or IMC, treatment results were variable based on red versus green light usage. Successful ablation was achieved in four out of six mucosal carcinoma and three out of four HGD patients who received red light. However, exposure to green light failed to achieve successful disease eradication or long-term remission. Significant complication, such as death, occurred after premature biopsy performance after treatment. This limited sample size study demonstrated that although mTHPC can destroy BE epithelium, the optimal light and drug dosimetry are still unknown.[43]

No randomized controlled prospective trials have been conducted to date comparing PDT with surgery for BE neoplasia management. However, a retrospective data analysis of HGD patients who received PDT (N = 129) or esophagectomy (N = 70) revealed no statistically significant differences in mortality or long-term survival based on choice of treatment modality.[44] The management of IMC with PDT seems to have a less efficacious profile, and thus cannot be uniformly recommended.

Major side effects of PDT include photosensitivity that requires patients to avoid postprocedure skin sunlight exposure, noncardiac chest pain, and symptomatic stricture formation. Risk factors for post-PDT stricture development include history of prior esophageal stricture, performance of EMR before PDT, and greater than one PDT treatment in a single session.[45] Development of subsquamous BE glands is another concern regarding PDT, because these glands may harbor neoplastic potential. However, the clinical significance of subsquamous BE glands is presently not fully understood. Reports of adenocarcinoma arising from subsquamous BE glands after PDT therapy have been described.[41,46] For these significant reasons, PDT usage has gone out of favor in recent years, with the advent of other available endoscopic ablative options.

RFA

Using either a balloon-based catheter or a focal device, RFA of BE tissue can be achieved in either a circumferential or localized fashion. Initially, a sizing balloon is inserted into the esophagus, and the optimal size of circumferential balloon is selected based on various pressure measurements in different esophageal locations. The process of RFA is a series of two separate applications of direct thermal energy with the electrodes imbedded in either the circumferential or focal device. Treated tissue is scraped between the first and second ablation to ensure adequate and uniform thermal contact. The most common complications associated with RFA include noncardiac chest pain, nontransmural lacerations, and a lower stricture rate when compared with EMR.

The efficacy and safety of RFA has been demonstrated in a gradual and progressive fashion. After initial thermal dose-escalation animal testing and preesophagectomy human experiments,[47,48] the first larger clinical study of RFA involved BE patients without dysplasia in the Ablation of Intestinal Metaplasia study from 2003 to 2005. This multicenter trial demonstrated a 70% complete remission of BE of the circumferentially treated group at 1-year follow up, without subsequent stricture formation or buried BE presence from 4306 biopsy fragments evaluated.[49] The subsequent Ablation of Intestinal Metaplasia II study reported 98% complete remission of IM after stepwise circumferential therapy with additional focal ablative therapy of remaining BE.[50]

RFA was also evaluated in 142 patients with BE HGD who demonstrated at 12-month follow-up complete remission of HGD in 90.2%, complete remission of dysplasia in 80.4%, and complete remission of IM in 54.3%.[51] In a recent landmark multicenter, sham-controlled trial, 127 patients with dysplastic BE were randomly assigned to receive either RFA or a sham procedure. Primary outcomes at 12 months included complete eradication of dysplasia and IM. In an intention-to-treat analyses, in LGD patients, complete eradication of dysplasia occurred in 90.5% from the ablation group, compared with only 22.7% from the control group ($P<.001$). In the HGD subgroup, complete eradication occurred in 81% of ablated patients, compared with 19% of the control group ($P<.001$). Overall, 77.4% of ablation patients demonstrated complete eradication of IM, in contrast to 2.3% of the control group ($P<.001$). There was less disease progression in patients from the ablation group (3.6% vs 16.3%; $P = .03$) and fewer cancers noted (1.2% vs 9.3%; $P = .045$). More reports of chest pain occurred after ablation than sham procedures, and a 6% esophageal stricture development rate was noted in the RFA treated group.[52] This markedly lower stricture rate associated with RFA as compared with EMR creates a significant advantage for RFA in the treatment of BE with flat HGD.

In the setting of BE with HGD, performance of EMR of any visible lesions with subsequent RFA of the remaining flat segment has been studied. Complete histologic eradication of all dysplasia and IM was achieved in 43 patients (98%). Postablation complications included mucosal laceration at prior EMR site (N = 3) and transient dysphagia (N = 4). No dysplasia recurred after a 21-month follow-up period.[53] A multicenter European trial involved EMR of visible lesions, followed by serial RFA. Focal escape endoscopic resection was used in cases of BE persistence despite RFA. The study included 24 patients, and eradication of neoplasia and IM was achieved in 95% and 88% of patients, respectively. These rates improved to 100% and 96%, respectively, after escape EMR in two patients. No neoplasia recurred within a median 22-month follow-up period.[54] Of note, neosquamous epithelium rigorous EMR and biopsy evaluation in a group of 22 post-RFA patients with baseline BE with IMC or HGD showed no evidence of persistent genetic abnormalities or buried BE glands.[55] To date, no published studies exist on outcomes of sole RFA therapy of BE with IMC.

Cryotherapy

The latest modality to arrive on the endoscopic horizon is cryotherapy. Sprayed liquid nitrogen is applied to the target area, and freeze-thaw cycles result in tissue destruction by intracellular disruption and tissue ischemia, with relative preservation of the extracellular matrix to promote less fibrosis formation.[56,57] Placement of an orogastric decompression tube allows for adequate excess nitrogen gas expulsion to help prevent inadvertent gastrointestinal viscus perforation. Repeat treatment sessions may be conducted every 4 to 6 weeks as needed to ensure complete remission of the target area's neoplasia.

In a prospective open-label trial, patients with BE and HGD or IMC who were deemed inoperable or who refused esophagectomy were enrolled for cryoablation. EMR was performed for pathologic staging of nodules before cryoablation and on focal residual areas during the follow-up period. Patients with prior ablation therapy were not excluded. Of 30 patients, 90% had pathologic downgrading postcryotherapy treatment. After a median follow-up of 1 year, elimination of cancer or downgrading of HGD was achieved in 80% of IMC and 68% of HGD patients, respectively. A perforation occurred in a patient with Marfan syndrome with a prototype system. Of six patients who showed a complete response, three had recurrence of dysplasia or cancer in the gastric cardia.[58]

Liquid nitrogen cryotherapy efficacy and safety profiles have been demonstrated in a four-center study of 24 patients (17 with HGD, 4 with IMC, and 3 with early stage adenocarcinoma). Complete response to HGD was found in 94% with HGD, and 100% with IMC and cancer. Complete response to IM was noted in 53% of HGD, 75% of IMC, and 67% with cancer. No symptoms were reported in 48% of 323 procedures. Three patient developed esophageal strictures, but all were successfully treated by dilation. Other complications included chest pain, dysphagia, sore throat, and the gastric perforation previously noted in the Marfan patient.[59]

In a more recent retrospective nonrandomized study involving nine centers over a 2-year treatment period, 98 patients with BE and HGD underwent 333 treatments. No esophageal perforations occurred, and esophageal strictures developed in three subjects. The efficacy analysis revealed a 97% complete eradication rate for HGD, 87% complete eradication of all dysplasia with persistent nondysplastic IM, and 57% had complete eradication of all IM.[60] Published results on efficacy of cryotherapy in treating BE with IMC are still awaited.

APPROACH TO A PATIENT WITH SUSPECTED BE NEOPLASIA

An expert gastrointestinal pathologist should confirm the diagnosis when neoplasia is diagnosed on an endoscopic biopsy (**Fig. 1**). A center with experience in BE may offer a multidisciplinary team of endoscopists, surgeons, and pathologists and a full range

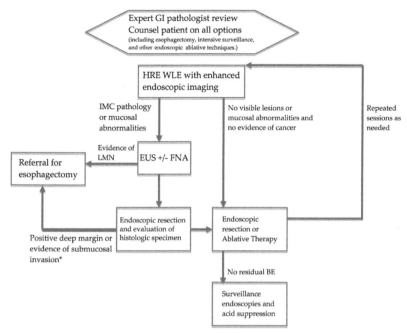

Fig. 1. Approach to a patient with BE with HGD and IMC.

of diagnostic and therapeutic modalities. Adherence to a rigorous and systematic endoscopic evaluation protocol must be followed to thoroughly investigate the entire Barrett's segment of neoplasia at all levels.[61] Patients should be thoroughly counseled on the risks and benefits of therapy and the appropriate alternate modalities or approaches.

Visible lesions in the setting of dysplasia carry a higher risk for harboring occult cancer than "flat" dysplasia.[62,63] Several studies have shown that visible lesions in the setting of HGD are associated with higher risk of occult submucosal invasion.[9,64,65] Careful white light examination is essential to identifying mucosal irregularities and visible lesions for targeted EMR.

Furthermore, a standardized criteria of endoscopic characterization of lesions is presented with the Paris classification. Protruding or depressed lesions are at higher risk for submucosal invasion than those slightly raised or flat areas.[64,65] Enhanced endoscopic imaging may be performed with supplementary additive technologies, such as narrow band imaging or endomicroscopy to further define more subtle mucosal irregularities that may harbor neoplasia. EMR provides an opportunity to stage the depth of a lesion in areas of question. In addition to these targeted biopsies and resection, a rigorous protocol with or without enhanced endoscopic imaging would allow for detection of occult neoplasia.

HGD obtained from multiple levels throughout a Barrett's segment has a higher risk of being associated with occult cancer.[65] Furthermore, in a risk analysis performed on patients with either HGD or IMC, multifocal neoplasia was cited as an independent risk factor for recurrence after endoscopic therapy. Additionally, in evaluations of specimens from endoscopic resection performed for Barrett's neoplasia, moderately or poorly differentiated cancers were associated with a higher incidence of submucosal invasion.[64,66] Risk factors for lymph node metastasis in esophageal adenocarcinoma are vascular invasion, lymphatic channel permutation, neural invasion, and grade of the tumor.[67,68]

Current controversies in the management of esophageal adenocarcinoma submucosal invasion still exist. A few recent studies show the risk of metastatic lymph node involvement is still significant despite subclassification of sm1 or sm2 to sm3 invasion.[37,38] Therefore, endoscopic management of adenocarcinoma invading into the submucosa cannot be uniformly recommended, and should be used only within a research protocol infrastructure for selected cases, in centers with expertise in endoscopic excision, and management of potential complications.

Endoscopic ultrasound has limitations in BE for differentiation between a T1a tumor (IMC) and a T1b (submucosal carcinoma) tumor, and EMR is allows for more accurate depth staging at this range.[69] However, given the risk of lymph node metastasis associated with IMC, EUS with fine-needle aspiration may identify patients with lymph node metastasis and therefore not eligible for endoscopic therapy.[70] EUS with or without fine-needle aspiration is a reasonable procedure in all patients with IMC and patients with visible lesions in the setting of HGD, who have a higher risk of occult cancer. Any patient demonstrating lymph node involvement should be referred for esophagectomy. The use of EUS in flat HGD may be questioned.[71]

Indications for esophagectomy include any evidence of lymph node metastasis, submucosal invasion, or involvement of the deep margin of an endoscopic resection. Patient characteristics, available endoscopic and surgical expertise, and endoscopic and histologic assessments of lesions need to be factored into decisions of suitability for endoscopic therapy.

If endoscopic therapy is pursued, treatment should be directed at treating the entire Barrett's epithelium with one or multiple modalities to achieve total Barrett's eradication to address risk of synchronous and metachronous lesion development. Endoscopic therapies to consider in the current management milieu include EMR or ablative therapies, such as PDT, RFA, or cryotherapy. Again, endoscopic resection of all mucosal irregularities provides an opportunity to accurately stage the lesion, eradicate the neoplasia, and gauge the need for further treatment. The remainder of the segment may be eradicated with endoscopic resection or ablative modalities. The combination of targeted EMR followed by RFA of the remainder of the segment enables balance of accurate diagnosis and staging, appropriate resection of higher-risk lesions, and mitigating the complication profile.

Lifelong surveillance with histologic sampling of the previously eradicated BE is currently required to monitor for recurrence of BE, the presence of buried glands, and the development of neoplasia. Suppression of acid may also decrease the risk of progression to dysplasia in patients with BE.[72] Endoscopic treatment is complemented by acid suppression therapy to prevent injury of the distal esophagus and to avoid recurrence of BE and progression to dysplasia.

SUMMARY

BE early neoplasia treatment has transitioned from radical esophagectomy to endoscopic organ-preserving options. The key to successful endoscopic management hinges on appropriate selection of patient candidates and critical detection of visible lesions through careful white light high-definition endoscopy with the possible assistance of endoscopic imaging techniques that may localize neoplasia. All visible lesions must be removed by EMR for definitive histopathologic staging. Total eradication of the entire BE segment must occur to protect against synchronous-metachronous lesion development.

The critical research issues that still remain unanswered for endoscopic BE management center on long-term survival and remission rates of both treated neoplasia and IM and further understanding of the pathogenesis in BE neoplasia. Elucidation of the genetic and molecular abnormalities on the development of BE and associated neoplasia might add to patient risk-stratification, rate of development and significance of buried BE glands, quality of life and cost assessments for the various modalities compared with standardized surgical cohorts, role of these therapies for LGD or non-dysplastic BE, and clinical impact of postendoscopic therapy surveillance.

It is increasingly evident that endoscopic management of BE neoplasia can be performed safely with comparable outcomes to that of surgery, sparing patients the added morbidity, mortality, and health care costs associated with operation. The development of endoscopic technologies and appropriate indications for treatment is currently evolving, and additional techniques and instruments are on the horizon. With this impressive contemporary evolution of the management of BE, the challenges faced by the field of gastrointestinal endoscopy are to validate these novel approaches, ensure adequate training, and continue to anticipate future clinical needs.

REFERENCES

1. Drewitz DJ, Sampliner RE, Garewal HS. The incidence of adenocarcinoma in Barrett's esophagus: a prospective study of 170 patients followed 4.8 years. Am J Gastroenterol 1997;92:212–5.
2. Hameeteman W, Tytgat GN, Houthoff HJ, et al. Barrett's esophagus: development of dysplasia and adenocarcinoma. Gastroenterology 1989;96:1249–56.
3. Shaheen NJ, Crosby MA, Bozymski EM, et al. Is there publication bias in the reporting of cancer risk in Barrett's esophagus? Gastroenterology 2000;119:333–8.
4. Haggitt RC. Pathology of Barrett's esophagus. J Gastrointest Surg 2000;4:117–8.
5. Gillison EW, Powell J, McConkey CC, et al. Surgical workload and outcome after resection for carcinoma of the oesophagus and cardia. Br J Surg 2002;89:344–8.
6. Liu JF, Wang QZ, Hou J. Surgical treatment for cancer of the oesophagus and gastric cardia in Hebei, China. Br J Surg 2004;91:90–8.
7. Ferguson MK, Naunheim KS. Resection for Barrett's mucosa with high-grade dysplasia: implications for prophylactic photodynamic therapy. J Thorac Cardiovasc Surg 1997;114:824–9.
8. Pellegrini CA, Pohl D. High-grade dysplasia in Barrett's esophagus: surveillance or operation? J Gastrointest Surg 2000;4:131–4.
9. Konda VJ, Ross AS, Ferguson MK, et al. Is the risk of concomitant invasive esophageal cancer in high-grade dysplasia in Barrett's esophagus overestimated? Clin Gastroenterol Hepatol 2008;6:159–64.
10. Pech O, Behrens A, May A, et al. Long-term results and risk factor analysis for recurrence after curative endoscopic therapy in 349 patients with high-grade intraepithelial neoplasia and mucosal adenocarcinoma in Barrett's oesophagus. Gut 2008;57:1200–6.
11. Birkmeyer JD, Siewers AE, Finlayson EV, et al. Hospital volume and surgical mortality in the United States. N Engl J Med 2002;346:1128–37.
12. Birkmeyer JD, Stukel TA, Siewers AE, et al. Surgeon volume and operative mortality in the United States. N Engl J Med 2003;349:2117–27.
13. Feith M, Stein HJ, Siewert JR. Pattern of lymphatic spread of Barrett's cancer. World J Surg 2003;27(9):1052–7.
14. Stein HJ, Feith M, Bruecher BL, et al. Early esophageal cancer: pattern of lymphatic spread and prognostic factors for long-term survival after surgical resection. Ann Surg 2005;242(4):566–73 [discussion: 73–5].

15. Holscher AH, Bollschweiler E, Schneider PM, et al. Early adenocarcinoma in Barrett's oesophagus. Br J Surg 1997;84(10):1470–3.

16. Siewert JR, Stein HJ, Feith M, et al. Histologic tumor type is an independent prognostic parameter in esophageal cancer: lessons from more than 1,000 consecutive resections at a single center in the Western world. Ann Surg 2001;234(3):360–7 [discussion: 368–9].

17. Rice TW, Zuccaro G Jr, Adelstein DJ, et al. Esophageal carcinoma: depth of tumor invasion is predictive of regional lymph node status. Ann Thorac Surg 1998;65(3):787–92.

18. van Sandick JW, van Lanschot JJ, ten Kate FJ, et al. Pathology of early invasive adenocarcinoma of the esophagus or esophagogastric junction: implications for therapeutic decision making. Cancer 2000;88(11):2429–37.

19. Wani S, Puli SR, Shaheen NJ, et al. Esophageal adenocarcinoma in Barrett's esophagus after endoscopic ablative therapy: a meta-analysis and systematic review. Am J Gastroenterol 2009;104:502–13.

20. Waxman I, Konda VJ. Mucosal ablation of Barrett esophagus. Nat Rev Gastroenterol Hepatol 2009;6:393–401.

21. Kantsevoy SV, Adler DG, Conway JD, et al. Endoscopic mucosal resection and endoscopic submucosal dissection. Gastrointest Endosc 2008;68:11–8.

22. Ell C, May A, Gossner L, et al. Endoscopic mucosal resection of early cancer and high-grade dysplasia in Barrett's esophagus. Gastroenterology 2000;118:670–7.

23. Nijhawan PK, Wang KK. Endoscopic mucosal resection for lesions with endoscopic features suggestive of malignancy and high-grade dysplasia within Barrett's esophagus. Gastrointest Endosc 2000;52:328–32.

24. Buttar NS, Wang KK, Lutzke LS, et al. Combined endoscopic mucosal resection and photodynamic therapy for esophageal neoplasia within Barrett's esophagus. Gastrointest Endosc 2001;54:682–8.

25. May A, Gossner L, Pech O, et al. Local endoscopic therapy for intraepithelial high-grade neoplasia and early adenocarcinoma in Barrett's oesophagus: acute-phase and intermediate results of a new treatment approach. Eur J Gastroenterol Hepatol 2002;14:1085–91.

26. May A, Gossner L, Pech O, et al. Intraepithelial high-grade neoplasia and early adenocarcinoma in short-segment Barrett's esophagus (SSBE): curative treatment using local endoscopic treatment techniques. Endoscopy 2002;34:604–10.

27. Pech O, May A, Gossner L, et al. Barrett's esophagus: endoscopic resection. Gastrointest Endosc Clin N Am 2003;13:505–12.

28. Larghi A, Lightdale CJ, Memeo L, et al. EUS followed by EMR for staging of high-grade dysplasia and early cancer in Barrett's esophagus. Gastrointest Endosc 2005;62:16–23.

29. Mino-Kenudson M, Brugge WR, Puricelli WP, et al. Management of superficial Barrett's epithelium-related neoplasms by endoscopic mucosal resection: clinicopathologic analysis of 27 cases. Am J Surg Pathol 2005;29:680–6.

30. Lopes CV, Hela M, Pesenti C, et al. Circumferential endoscopic resection of Barrett's esophagus with high-grade dysplasia or early adenocarcinoma. Surg Endosc 2007;21:820–4.

31. Chennat J, Konda VJ, Ross AS, et al. Complete Barrett's eradication endoscopic mucosal resection: an effective treatment modality for high-grade dysplasia and intramucosal carcinoma: an American single-center experience. Am J Gastroenterol 2009;104:2684–92.

32. Seewald S, Akaraviputh T, Seitz U, et al. Circumferential EMR and complete removal of Barrett's epithelium: a new approach to management of Barrett's

esophagus containing high-grade intraepithelial neoplasia and intramucosal carcinoma. Gastrointest Endosc 2003;57:854–9.

33. Peters FP, Kara MA, Rosmolen WD, et al. Stepwise radical endoscopic resection is effective for complete removal of Barrett's esophagus with early neoplasia: a prospective study. Am J Gastroenterol 2006;101:1449–57.

34. Seewald S, Ang TL, Gotoda T, et al. Total endoscopic resection of Barrett esophagus. Endoscopy 2008;40:1016–20.

35. Yoshinaga S, Gotoda T, Kusano C, et al. Clinical impact of endoscopic submucosal dissection for superficial adenocarcinoma located at the esophagogastric junction. Gastrointest Endosc 2008;67:202–9.

36. Manner H, May A, Pech O, et al. Early Barrett's carcinoma with "low-risk" submucosal invasion: long-term results of endoscopic resection with a curative intent. Am J Gastroenterol 2008;103:2589–97.

37. Badreddine RJ, Prasad GA, Lewis JT, et al. Depth of submucosal invasion does not predict lymph node metastasis and survival of patients with esophageal carcinoma. Clin Gastroenterol Hepatol 2010;8(3):248–53.

38. Sepesi B, Watson TJ, Zhou D, et al. Are endoscopic therapies appropriate for superficial submucosal esophageal adenocarcinoma? An analysis of esophagectomy specimens. J Am Coll Surg 2010;210(4):418–27.

39. Gross SA, Wolfsen HC. The role of photodynamic therapy in the esophagus. Gastrointest Endosc Clin N Am 2010;20(1):35–53.

40. Overholt BF, Wang KK, Burdick JS, et al. Five-year efficacy and safety of photodynamic therapy with photofrin in Barrett's high-grade dysplasia. Gastrointest Endosc 2007;66:460–8.

41. Overholt BF, Panjehpour M, Halberg DL. Photodynamic therapy for Barrett's esophagus with dysplasia and/or early stage carcinoma: long-term results. Gastrointest Endosc 2003;58:183–8.

42. Pech O, Gossner L, May A, et al. Long-term results of photodynamic therapy with 5-aminolevulinic acid for superficial Barrett's cancer and high-grade intraepithelial neoplasia. Gastrointest Endosc 2005;62:24–30.

43. Lovat LB, Jamieson NF, Novelli MR, et al. Photodynamic therapy with m-tetrahydroxyphenyl chlorin for high-grade dysplasia and early cancer in Barrett's columnar lined esophagus. Gastrointest Endosc 2005;62:617–23.

44. Prasad GA, Wang KK, Buttar NS, et al. Long-term survival following endoscopic and surgical treatment of high-grade dysplasia in Barrett's esophagus. Gastroenterology 2007;132:1226–33.

45. Prasad GA, Wang KK, Buttar NS, et al. Predictors of stricture formation after photodynamic therapy for high-grade dysplasia in Barrett's esophagus. Gastrointest Endosc 2007;65:60–6.

46. Van Laethem JL, Peny MO, Salmon I, et al. Intramucosal adenocarcinoma arising under squamous re-epithelialisation of Barrett's oesophagus. Gut 2000;46:574–7.

47. Dunkin BJ, Martinez J, Bejarano PA, et al. Thin-layer ablation of human esophageal epithelium using a bipolar radiofrequency balloon device. Surg Endosc 2006;20:125–30.

48. Ganz RA, Utley DS, Stern RA, et al. Complete ablation of esophageal epithelium with a balloon-based bipolar electrode: a phased evaluation in the porcine and in the human esophagus. Gastrointest Endosc 2004;60:1002–10.

49. Sharma VK, Wang KK, Overholt BF, et al. Balloon-based, circumferential, endoscopic radiofrequency ablation of Barrett's esophagus: 1-year follow-up of 100 patients. Gastrointest Endosc 2007;65:185–95.

50. Fleischer DE, Overholt BF, Sharma VK, et al. Endoscopic ablation of Barrett's esophagus: a multicenter study with 2.5-year follow-up. Gastrointest Endosc 2008;68:867–76.

51. Ganz RA, Overholt BF, Sharma VK, et al. Circumferential ablation of Barrett's esophagus that contains high-grade dysplasia: a U.S. multicenter registry. Gastrointest Endosc 2008;68:35–40.

52. Shaheen NJ, Sharma P, Overholt BF, et al. Radiofrequency ablation in Barrett's esophagus with dysplasia. N Engl J Med 2009;360:2277–88.

53. Pouw RE, Gondrie JJ, Sondermeijer CM, et al. Eradication of Barrett esophagus with early neoplasia by radiofrequency ablation, with or without endoscopic resection. J Gastrointest Surg 2008;12:1627–36 [discussion: 1636–7].

54. Pouw RE, Wirths K, Eisendrath P, et al. Efficacy of radiofrequency ablation combined with endoscopic resection for Barrett's esophagus with early neoplasia. Clin Gastroenterol Hepatol 2010;8(1):23–9.

55. Pouw RE, Gondrie JJ, Rygiel AM, et al. Properties of the neosquamous epithelium after radiofrequency ablation of Barrett's esophagus containing neoplasia. Am J Gastroenterol 2009;104:1366–73.

56. Kuflik EG. Cryosurgery updated. J Am Acad Dermatol 1994;31:925–44 [quiz: 944–6].

57. Wynn TA. Common and unique mechanisms regulate fibrosis in various fibroproliferative diseases. J Clin Invest 2007;117:524–9.

58. Dumot JA, Vargo JJII, Falk GW, et al. An open-label, prospective trial of cryospray ablation for Barrett's esophagus high-grade dysplasia and early esophageal cancer in high-risk patients. Gastrointest Endosc 2009;70:635–44.

59. Greenwald BD, Dumot JA, Horwhat JD, et al. Safety, tolerability, and efficacy of endoscopic low-pressure liquid nitrogen spray cryotherapy in the esophagus. Dis Esophagus 2010;23(1):13–9.

60. Shaheen NJ, Greenwald BD, Peery AF, et al. Safety and efficacy of endoscopic spray cryotherapy for Barrett's esophagus with high-grade dysplasia. Gastrointest Endosc 2010;71(4):680–5.

61. Curvers WL, Bansal A, Sharma P, et al. Endoscopic work-up of early Barrett's neoplasia. Endoscopy 2008;40:1000–7.

62. Nigro JJ, Hagen JA, DeMeester TR, et al. Occult esophageal adenocarcinoma: extent of disease and implications for effective therapy. Ann Surg 1999;230: 433–8 [discussion: 438–40].

63. Tharavej C, Hagen JA, Peters JH, et al. Predictive factors of coexisting cancer in Barrett's high-grade dysplasia. Surg Endosc 2006;20:439–43.

64. Peters FP, Brakenhoff KP, Curvers WL, et al. Histologic evaluation of resection specimens obtained at 293 endoscopic resections in Barrett's esophagus. Gastrointest Endosc 2008;67:604–9.

65. Endoscopic Classification Review Group. Update on the Paris classification of superficial neoplastic lesions in the digestive tract. Endoscopy 2005;37:570–8.

66. Vieth M, Ell C, Gossner L, et al. Histological analysis of endoscopic resection specimens from 326 patients with Barrett's esophagus and early neoplasia. Endoscopy 2004;36:776–81.

67. Ancona E, Rampado S, Cassaro M, et al. Prediction of lymph node status in superficial esophageal carcinoma. Ann Surg Oncol 2008;15:3278–88.

68. Gockel I, Domeyer M, Sgourakis GG, et al. Prediction model of lymph node metastasis in superficial esophageal adenocarcinoma and squamous cell cancer including D2-40 immunostaining. J Surg Oncol 2009;100:191–8.

69. Pech O, Gunter E, Ell C. Endosonography of high-grade intra-epithelial neoplasia/ early cancer. Best Pract Res Clin Gastroenterol 2009;23:639–47.
70. Shami VM, Villaverde A, Stearns L, et al. Clinical impact of conventional endoso-nography and endoscopic ultrasound-guided fine-needle aspiration in the assessment of patients with Barrett's esophagus and high-grade dysplasia or in-tramucosal carcinoma who have been referred for endoscopic ablation therapy. Endoscopy 2006;38:157–61.
71. Thomas T, Gilbert D, Kaye PV, et al. High-resolution endoscopy and endoscopic ultrasound for evaluation of early neoplasia in Barrett's esophagus. Surg Endosc 2010;24:1110–6.
72. El-Serag HB, Aguirre TV, Davis S, et al. Proton pump inhibitors are associated with reduced incidence of dysplasia in Barrett's esophagus. Am J Gastroenterol 2004;99:1877–83.

Role of Minimally Invasive Surgery in the Modern Treatment of Barrett's Esophagus

Marco G. Patti, MD[a],*, Fernando A.M. Herbella, MD[b]

KEYWORDS

- Gastroesophageal reflux disease • Barrett's esophagus
- Radiofrequency ablation • Endoscopic mucosal resection
- Adenocarcinoma of the esophagus
- Laparoscopic fundoplication • Esophagectomy

Gastroesophageal reflux disease (GERD) is a highly prevalent disease. Population studies have demonstrated that a significant proportion of individuals experience GERD symptoms weekly.[1,2] Barrett's esophagus (BE), defined by the presence of intestinal metaplasia (columnar epithelium with goblet cells), is considered a consequence of chronic reflux.[3] The real prevalence of BE is unknown because (1) there are no clinical manifestations of BE per se, so the symptoms alone cannot distinguish between GERD and GERD with BE[4]; (2) some patients with BE are asymptomatic[5]; and (3) the definition of BE has changed with time.[6,7] Different studies show a variable prevalence of BE according to the sampled population, which consists of normal individuals, patients with reflux symptoms, or individuals who had an upper endoscopy for evaluation of symptoms not related to reflux. In a random sample of 3000 adults in Sweden who underwent endoscopy with biopsies, a prevalence of BE of 1.6% was reported.[5] A similar prevalence was found in Italian and Chinese studies.[8,9] This rate increases 3-fold in upper endoscopy series[10,11] and increases 10 times if only patients with chronic GERD are considered.[12]

Through a sequence of events, the metaplastic epithelium can evolve to low-grade dysplasia, high-grade dysplasia (HGD), and eventually esophageal adenocarcinoma

Disclosure: The authors have nothing to disclose.
[a] Department of Surgery, University of Chicago, 5841 South Maryland Avenue, Room G-201, Chicago, IL 60637, USA
[b] Department of Surgery, University of Chicago, 5841 South Maryland Avenue, Room G-201, Chicago, IL 60637, USA
* Corresponding author.
E-mail address: mpatti@surgery.bsd.uchicago.edu

(EAC). The incidence of EAC has increased 8-fold in the last 30 years, and this increase is thought to be secondary to GERD through the development of BE.[13]

The last decade has witnessed a radical change in the therapeutic approach to BE. In the past, the focus of treatment was on control of reflux with the goal of causing regression or stopping the progression to cancer, whereas today the focus is on ablation of the BE epithelium with regeneration of normal squamous epithelium. This goal can be achieved with the use of new endoscopic treatment modalities that are safe and effective and may eventually alter the natural history of this disease by interrupting the cascade of events that lead to cancer.

This review defines the role of surgery in the modern treatment of BE, taking into consideration the pathophysiology of the disease and the new endoscopic procedures available at present.

PATHOPHYSIOLOGY OF BE: IMPLICATIONS FOR TREATMENT

GERD is a multifactorial disease.[14] The normal physiologic mechanism that protects the esophagus from reflux is based on the interaction of multiple factors, such as the pressure, length, and behavior of the lower esophageal sphincter (LES); the synergistic action of the diaphragm; and the effectiveness of esophageal peristalsis. These factors work in concert to limit the amount of reflux of gastric contents into the esophagus to a physiologic level, avoiding the development of symptoms and mucosal injury. In BE, this synergism is altered because a pan-esophageal motor disorder is frequently present.

LES

Physiologically, the LES is a 3- to 4-cm long segment of tonically contracted smooth muscle.[15] An effective LES must have an adequate total and intra-abdominal length and an adequate resting pressure.[16] However, a normal LES pressure does not exclude GERD, because abnormal transient relaxations may occur. Periodic relaxations of the LES in normal individuals have been termed transient LES relaxations (TLESRs) to distinguish them from relaxations triggered by swallowing. TLESRs account for the physiologic reflux found in normal subjects. However, when TLESRs become more frequent and prolonged, they can contribute to the development of GERD, and this phenomenon seems to explain the reflux observed in about 40% of patients with GERD whose resting LES pressure is normal. The cause of TLESRs is unknown, but postprandial gastric distention is probably involved.[17] It seems that TLESRs play a role in patients with no mucosal injury or low grades of esophagitis, whereas a mechanically incompetent LES (short and hypotensive) is more often associated with worse mucosal damage such as in BE.[18]

Medical treatment has been traditionally directed toward the decrease of acid production. At present, the focus is on medications that can affect the LES. For instance, initial studies with lesogaberan, a γ-aminobutyric acid type B receptor agonist, have shown a decreased number of TLESRs and reflux episodes and an increased LES pressure.[17] These data underline that an incompetent LES represents a permanent defect of the gastroesophageal barrier. It is well proven that a fundoplication can correct the functional and mechanical profile of the LES, resulting in the control of any type of reflux from the stomach into the esophagus.

Peristalsis

Esophageal peristalsis is an important component of the antireflux mechanism because it is the main determinant of esophageal clearance of the gastric refluxate.

Defective peristalsis is associated with more severe GERD, both in terms of symptoms and mucosal damage.[19]

It is known that 40% to 50% of patients with GERD have abnormal peristalsis.[19] This dysmotility is particularly severe in about 20% of patients because of very low amplitude of peristalsis and/or abnormal propagation of the peristaltic waves (ineffective esophageal motility). Because esophageal clearance is slower when peristalsis is ineffective, the refluxate is in contact with the esophageal mucosa for a longer period and is able to reach the upper esophagus and pharynx more often. Thus, these patients are prone to more severe mucosal injury (including BE) and more frequent extraesophageal symptoms such as cough or hoarseness.[19]

It is still unclear whether esophageal dysmotility is a primary condition leading to GERD or a consequence of esophageal inflammation. Medical therapy does not ameliorate esophageal peristalsis.[20] However, it has been shown that an effective fundoplication often improves abnormal peristalsis, suggesting that the dysmotility in most patients is the consequence rather than the cause of abnormal reflux.[21]

Diaphragm

The LES and the diaphragmatic crura work together to form a sphincter, in which the smooth muscle of the LES coordinates with the striated muscle of the diaphragm to protect against reflux. The pinchcock action of the diaphragm is particularly important as protection against reflux induced by sudden increases in intra-abdominal pressure, such as during coughing and bending. This mechanism is disrupted by the presence and size of the hiatal hernia. It has been shown that in patients with a large hiatal hernia (>5 cm), the LES is shorter and weaker, the amount of reflux is greater, and the acid clearance is slower. As a consequence, the degree of mucosal injury is greater.[22,23] The presence of a hiatal hernia has been associated with early recurrence and failure of medical therapy for GERD.[23] On the other end, the reduction of a hiatal hernia with the narrowing of the esophageal hiatus is a key element in the performance of a fundoplication.

In a study of 502 consecutive patients with GERD (documented by pH monitoring), Campos and colleagues[24] identified 3 factors that predicted the presence of BE: (1) a hiatal hernia measuring more than 4 cm, (2) an incompetent LES, and (3) long reflux episodes. This study suggests that there is a more severe compromise of the antireflux mechanism in patients with BE. These abnormalities can be corrected by a properly constructed fundoplication.

The Refluxate

Gastric and duodenal contents play a role in the development of GERD. Today, it is recognized that bile salts and pancreatic enzymes are part of the refluxate and are injurious to the esophageal mucosa. The definitive proof that bile reflux contributes to the pathogenesis of GERD was possible with the Bilitec 2000 (Medtronic, Minneapolis, MN, USA), which uses bilirubin as a marker for duodenal reflux. In a seminal study from the University of Southern California, Kauer and colleagues[25] demonstrated that 58% of patients with GERD had mixed reflux, with increased esophageal exposure to gastric and duodenal juices. In addition, patients with Barrett metaplasia had a higher prevalence of abnormal esophageal bilirubin exposure than those with erosive esophagitis or no injury. In a subsequent study involving a large cohort of patients, the investigators showed that reflux of bile was the leading factor associated with BE and early cancer and that it can be suppressed by a fundoplication but not by acid suppression alone.[26]

Implications For Treatment

Acid-reducing medications or a laparoscopic fundoplication are used today for the treatment of GERD. Treatment with proton pump inhibitors (PPIs) has the following major limitations:

- As shown by pH-impedance monitoring, PPIs only change the pH of the gastric refluxate, not the occurrence and the number of reflux episodes, through a functionally or mechanically incompetent LES.[27]
- The duodenal components of the refluxate are unaffected by PPI treatment.[26]
- When pH monitoring is performed in patients with Barrett metaplasia who are asymptomatic during PPI treatment, about 40% to 80% of them still have abnormal acid reflux.[28,29]

On the other hand, a fundoplication controls any type of reflux. The operation is effective because it improves esophageal motility, both in terms of LES competence and quality of esophageal peristalsis.[21] Control of reflux is not influenced by the pattern of reflux, being equally effective when reflux is upright, supine, or bipositional.[30] In addition, the operation is equally safe and effective in young or elderly patients.[31]

A fundoplication can be done laparoscopically with a short hospital stay, minimal postoperative discomfort, fast recovery time, and excellent results. Long-term studies have shown that laparoscopic fundoplication controls symptoms in about 90% of patients after 10 years.[32]

The role of surgery in the modern treatment of GERD and BE is reviewed step by step, from symptoms to metaplasia and from HGD to EAC.

GERD and Symptoms

PPIs or antireflux surgery is the option available for the treatment of GERD. Surgery is indicated in the following circumstances:

- When symptoms (heartburn and especially regurgitation) are not completely controlled by medical treatment
- When it is thought that respiratory symptoms are induced by gastroesophageal reflux. Mainie and colleagues[33] have shown that a laparoscopic Nissen fundoplication is the treatment of choice in patients resistant to PPIs, in whom nonacid or acid reflux is demonstrated by multichannel intraluminal pH-impedance monitoring, and in those with a positive symptom index
- Poor patient compliance
- High cost of medical therapy
- Postmenopausal women with osteoporosis. PPIs and histamine2 receptor antagonists increase the risk of hip and femur fractures[34]
- Young and symptomatic patients for whom lifelong medical treatment is not advisable.

Based on the data present in the literature, there is no definitive evidence that one form of treatment is better than the other in preventing progression to Barrett metaplasia. However, few studies seem to suggest that an antireflux operation might be more effective than medical treatment. Using endoscopy, Oberg and colleagues[35] studied 69 patients with reflux symptoms but no metaplasia; 49 were treated with chronic acid suppression therapy and 20 underwent a fundoplication (19 with normalization of the acid reflux as determined by postoperative pH monitoring). The investigators showed that surgery was associated with a 10-fold decreased chance of developing intestinal metaplasia.[35] Similar findings were reported by Wetscher and colleagues[36] in a prospective study of patients with GERD who were treated either medically (83 patients with PPIs and cisapride) or by a fundoplication (42 patients). Barrett metaplasia developed in 14.5% of patients treated medically (median follow-up, 2 years) but in none of the patients treated surgically (median follow-up, 3.5 years).[36] These results seem to suggest that antireflux surgery is more effective than acid suppression, probably because it restores the LES competence and stops any type of reflux, acid or bilious.

Metaplasia

About 10% to 15% of patients with GERD (proved by pH monitoring) eventually develop metaplasia.[37] Long duration of symptoms, a large hiatal hernia, an incompetent LES, and the presence of acid and bile reflux are considered potential risk factors for the progression from symptoms to metaplasia. It is controversial whether medical or surgical treatment can cause regression and affect the natural history of the disease. However, it seems that a fundoplication causes regression to nonmetaplastic epithelium in 30% to 60% of patients with a short-segment BE (SSBE, <3 cm).[38,39] For instance, Oelschlager and colleagues[38] studied the effect of laparoscopic antireflux surgery in 106 consecutive patients with BE. Heartburn resolved or improved in 96% of patients and regurgitation in 84%. Among 90 patients who had endoscopic follow-up, 54 had an SSBE and 36 had a long-segment BE (LSBE). Postoperative endoscopy and pathology revealed complete regression of intestinal metaplasia in 56% of patients with SSBE but in none with an LSBE. One of the patients with LSBE developed an adenocarcinoma within 10 months of operation.[38] Bowers and colleagues[39] demonstrated loss of intestinal metaplasia in the tubular esophagus in 47% of patients after a fundoplication. None of the patients developed HGD or adenocarcinoma during follow-up. About 97% of patients were satisfied with the results of the operation.

In summary, it seems that antireflux surgery is effective in symptom control in patients with BE and that it can cause regression when SSBE, but not LSBE, is present. Based on these data and the understanding of the pathophysiology of the disease, the authors propose that patients should be treated initially with radiofrequency ablation (RFA) to eliminate the metaplastic epithelium and subsequently have a fundoplication. Even though most of the protocols currently in place use PPI therapy after RFA, this approach is not useful for the following reasons:

- Pathophysiology of GERD, as previously described. PPIs do not affect the overall occurrence of reflux and do not improve the abnormal motility.
- Some patients develop metaplasia while being treated with PPIs.
- RFA does not alter the genetic or environmental causes of GERD.

There is some concern about the side effects of an antireflux operation and the long-term results. Referral of these patients to centers where proven expertise is present is recommended. Although the concept of outcome linked to volume is now accepted for high-risk operations, such as esophagectomy for cancer, it is not equally established for benign esophageal diseases.[40,41] For operations such as antireflux surgery, the expertise of the team managing these patients, particularly the surgeon's experience, is of key importance in the performance of a safe, effective, and long-lasting laparoscopic fundoplication.

Low-Grade Dysplasia

For patients with low-grade dysplasia, the same therapeutic approach as that for patients with metaplasia is recommended. However, after the initial endoscopy, patients should be treated for about 8 weeks with high doses of PPI and subsequently have a repeat endoscopy. Once the inflammation is resolved, it is easier for the pathologist to determine if the patient has metaplasia, low-grade dysplasia, or HGD.

HGD and Adenocarcinoma

The introduction of new endoscopic techniques such as RFA and endoscopic mucosal resection (EMR) has revolutionized the treatment of BE associated with HGD and early EAC,[42,43] obviating an esophagectomy in most patients with these conditions.

In the past, the presence of HGD and early EAC was usually considered as an indication for esophagectomy. This recommendation was based on the following 2 considerations:

1. Progression of the disease. Many studies had shown a high rate of progression from HGD to EAC, of about 50% at 5 years and 80% at 8 years.[44,45]
2. It was believed that in about 40% of patients in whom an esophagectomy was performed for HGD, an invasive adenocarcinoma was instead found in the resected specimen.[46]

However, most of these studies had major flaws. In most patients, the diagnosis was based on an endoscopy with random biopsies only. If a more rigid protocol (4-quadrant biopsies every cm) had been used, an EAC would have been detected preoperatively in many patients. In addition, often a second pathologist did not review the slides of the endoscopic biopsies. This review process is important because of the difficulty in distinguishing between HGD and a superficial cancer and the existence of well-known interobserver variation.[47] Had these procedures been properly done, the 40% rate of EAC found in the resected specimen would have been much lower.

Although in the past the differentiation between HGD and superficial cancer was often a moot point because a resection was ultimately performed, it is of paramount importance today because of the use of RFA and EMR. HGD (carcinoma in situ) is a neoplastic process without invasion of the basement membrane. According to the American Joint Commission on Cancer, an intramucosal carcinoma (IMC) or T1a is a tumor limited to the lamina propria and a submucosal carcinoma or T1b is a tumor that has invaded past the muscularis mucosae, which is considered an invasive adenocarcinoma (IEAC). Each stage has a different risk of lymph node metastases; it is 0% for HGD, around 7% for a T1a cancer, and about 25% for a T1b cancer.[48]

In a recent study, Konda and colleagues[46] reviewed reports of patients who had esophagectomy for HGD in BE to determine the true incidence of IEAC. Although the overall rate was around 40%, it decreased to 12.7% when studies that differentiated between intramucosal and submucosal invasion were considered. Differentiating between IMC (T1a) and IEAC (T1b and beyond) is of paramount importance because HGD and IMC can be treated endoscopically in most cases, thereby restricting esophageal resection to a small subset of patients. When there is a need to distinguish between T1a and T1b, EMR is useful as a diagnostic and staging procedure. EMR is important in the case of visible lesions in the setting of HGD because they are associated with a higher risk of IEAC.

Based on these considerations, the patients in whom an esophagectomy should still be considered can be determined as follows:

- Patients in whom lymph node involvement is clearly shown by endoscopic ultrasonography (EUS)-guided fine-needle aspiration, even if it is an IMC.

- Patients who are young. Surveillance for 20 to 40 years is not a viable and reasonable option because of the risk of losing patients to follow-up, with some of them coming back with dysphagia caused by advanced cancer.
- Patients who are not willing or cannot afford the rigorous follow-up associated with endoscopic treatment. For instance, in the Wiesbaden experience, patients underwent intensive staging with EUS, high-resolution videoendoscopy, and a rigid biopsy protocol with review by 2 different pathologists. After treatment, patients had follow-up endoscopy at 1, 2, 3, 6, 9, 12, 16, 24, 30, and 36 months, again with high-resolution chromoendoscopy, computed tomography, EUS, and multiple biopsies.[42] It seems reasonable to assume that many patients would not be compliant over time and that after 3 to 5 years the dropout rate could be high.
- Patients with multifocal disease and a LSBE. In these patients, there is the risk of missing synchronous or metachronous lesions.[49]
- Patients in whom BE is still present after RFA and/or EMR. The risk of developing an IEAC in the remaining BE epithelium is quite high. In a study of 261 patients with dysplasia or IMC, Badreddine and colleagues[50] found that significant predictors of recurrence on a multivariate model were history of smoking, old age, and presence of residual nondysplastic BE. Recurrence occurred in 47 of 261 (17%) patients treated with photodynamic therapy, with or without EMR. LSBE (7 and 10 cm) was present before ablation in 2 patients with recurring adenocarcinoma.
- Patients who are healthy and do not want to have a lifelong and rigid follow-up or who are concerned about developing an IEAC.

Even though it is recognized that an esophagectomy is curative because it removes all the BE, there is still concern about the mortality rate of the operation and the quality of life afterward. There is a major difference between resections done for advanced esophageal cancer and those performed for T1 lesions. Many series have, in fact, shown that the mortality rate for early cancer is close to 0% and that after the immediate postoperative period, the quality of life is excellent.[48,51] For instance, the Luketich group has shown that esophagectomy for T1 lesions can be done with a 0% mortality rate.[48] In addition, the use of minimally invasive techniques has brought an improvement in the immediate postoperative course because it is associated with less postoperative pain, a shorter hospital stay, and a faster recovery time.[48] Chang and colleagues[51] showed that postoperative symptoms caused by esophagectomy are common but mild and do not interfere with the quality of life, which is excellent and similar to that of the general population.

SUMMARY

The authors recommend that patients with BE be treated in centers with known expertise and where a multidisciplinary approach is used. Treatment should be individualized, taking into account the disease process, the patient's characteristics and logistics, and the available endoscopic and surgical expertise.

REFERENCES

1. Moayyedi P, Axon AT. Review article: gastro-oesophageal reflux disease–the extent of the problem. Aliment Pharmacol Ther 2005;22:11–9.
2. Moraes-Filho JP, Chinzon D, Eisig JN, et al. Prevalence of heartburn and gastroesophageal reflux disease in the urban Brazilian population. Arq Gastroenterol 2005;42:122–7.

3. Reid BJ, Li X, Galipeau PC, et al. Barrett's oesophagus and oesophageal adeno-carcinoma: time for a new synthesis. Nat Rev Cancer 2010;10:87–101.

4. Lord RV, DeMeester SR, Peters JH, et al. Hiatal hernia, lower esophageal sphincter incompetence, and effectiveness of Nissen fundoplication in the spectrum of gastroesophageal reflux disease. J Gastrointest Surg 2009;13:602–10.

5. Ronkainen J, Aro P, Storskrubb T, et al. Prevalence of Barrett's esophagus in the general population: an endoscopic study. Gastroenterology 2005;129:1825–31.

6. DeMeester SR, DeMeester TR. Columnar mucosa and intestinal metaplasia of the esophagus: fifty years of controversy. Ann Surg 2000;231:303–21.

7. Herbella FA, Matone J, Del Grande JC. Eponyms in esophageal surgery, part 2. Dis Esophagus 2005;18:4–16.

8. Zagari RM, Fuccio L, Wallander, et al. Gastro-oesophageal reflux symptoms, oesophagitis and Barrett's oesophagus in the general population: the Loiano-Monghidoro study. Gut 2008;57:1354–9.

9. Peng S, Cui Y, Xiao YL, et al. Prevalence of erosive esophagitis and Barrett's esophagus in the adult Chinese population. Endoscopy 2009;41:1011–7.

10. Rex DK, Cummings OW, Shaw M, et al. Screening for Barrett's esophagus in colonoscopy patients with and without heartburn. Gastroenterology 2003;125: 1670–7.

11. Kim JY, Kim YS, Jung MK, et al. Prevalence of Barrett's esophagus in Korea. J Gastroenterol Hepatol 2005;20:633–6.

12. Westhoff B, Brotze S, Weston A, et al. The frequency of Barrett's esophagus in high-risk patients with chronic GERD. Gastrointest Endosc 2005;61:226–31.

13. Pohl H, Sirovich B, Welch HG. Esophageal adenocarcinoma incidence: are we reaching the peak? Cancer Epidemiol Biomarkers Prev 2010;19:1468–70.

14. Herbella FA, Patti MG. Gastroesophageal reflux disease: from pathophysiology to treatment. World J Gastroenterol 2010;16:3745–9.

15. Kahrilas PJ. Anatomy and physiology of the gastroesophageal junction. Gastroenterol Clin North Am 1997;26:467–86.

16. Zaninotto G, DeMeester TR, Schwizer W, et al. The lower esophageal sphincter in health and disease. Am J Surg 1988;155:104–11.

17. Boeckxtaens GE, Beaumont H, Mertens V, et al. Effect of lesogaberan on reflux and lower esophageal sphincter function in patients with gastroesophageal reflux disease. Gastroenterology 2010;139:409–17.

18. Stein HJ, Barlow AP, DeMeester TR, et al. Complications of gastroesophageal reflux disease. Role of the lower esophageal sphincter, esophageal acid and acid/alkaline exposure, and duodenogastric reflux. Ann Surg 1992;216:35–43.

19. Diener U, Patti MG, Molena D, et al. Esophageal dysmotility and gastroesophageal reflux disease. J Gastrointest Surg 2001;5:260–5.

20. Xu JY, Xie XP, Song GQ, et al. Healing of severe reflux esophagitis with PPI does not improve esophageal dysmotility. Dis Esophagus 2007;20:346–52.

21. Herbella FA, Tedesco P, Nipomnick I, et al. Effect of partial and total laparoscopic fundoplication on esophageal body motility. Surg Endosc 2007;21:285–8.

22. Patti MG, Goldberg HI, Arcerito M, et al. Hiatal hernia size affects lower esophageal sphincter function, esophageal acid exposure, and the degree of mucosal injury. Am J Surg 1996;171:182–6.

23. Gordon C, Kang JY, Neild PJ, et al. The role of the hiatus hernia in gastro-oesophageal reflux disease. Aliment Pharmacol Ther 2004;20:719–32.

24. Campos GM, Peters JH, DeMeester TR, et al. Predictive factors of Barrett's esophagus: multivariate analysis of 502 patients with gastroesophageal reflux disease. Arch Surg 2001;136:1267–73.

25. Kauer WK, Peters JH, DeMeester TR, et al. Mixed reflux of gastric and duodenal juice is more harmful to the esophagus than gastric juice alone. The need for surgical therapy re-emphasized. Ann Surg 1995;222:525–31.

26. Stein HJ, Kauer WK, Feussner H, et al. Bile reflux in benign and malignant Barrett's esophagus: effect of medical acid suppression and Nissen fundoplication. J Gastrointest Surg 1998;4:333–41.

27. Tamhankar AP, Peters JH, Portale G, et al. Omeprazole does not reduce gastro-esophageal reflux: new insights using multichannel intraluminal impedance technology. J Gastrointest Surg 2004;8:890–7.

28. Katzka DA, Castell DO. Successful elimination of reflux symptoms does not insure adequate control of acid reflux in patients with Barrett's esophagus. Am J Gastroenterol 1994;89:989–91.

29. Ouatu-Lascar R, Triadafilopoulos G. Complete elimination of reflux symptoms does not guarantee normalization of intra-esophageal acid reflux in patients with Barrett's esophagus. Am J Gastroenterol 1998;93:711–6.

30. Meneghetti AT, Tedesco P, Galvani C, et al. Outcomes after laparoscopic Nissen fundoplication are not influenced by the pattern of reflux. Dis Esophagus 2008; 21:165–9.

31. Tedesco P, Lobo E, Way LW, et al. Laparoscopic fundoplication in elderly patients with gastroesophageal reflux disease. Arch Surg 2006;141:289–92.

32. Dallemagne B, Weerts J, Markiewicz S, et al. Clinical results of laparoscopic fundoplication at 10 years after surgery. Surg Endosc 2006;20:159–65.

33. Mainie I, Tutuian R, Agrawal A, et al. Combined multichannel impedance-pH monitoring to select patients with persistent gastro-oesophageal reflux for laparoscopic fundoplication. Br J Surg 2006;93:1483–7.

34. Corley DA, Kubo A, Zhao W, et al. Proton pump inhibitors and histamine-2 receptor antagonists are associated with hip fractures among at-risk patients. Gastroenterology 2010;139:93–101.

35. Oberg S, Johansson J, Wenner J, et al. Endoscopic surveillance of columnar liner esophagus. Frequency of intestinal metaplasia detection and impact of antireflux surgery. Ann Surg 2001;234:619–26.

36. Wetscher GJ, Gadenstaetter M, Klingler PJ, et al. Efficacy of medical therapy and antireflux surgery to prevent Barrett's metaplasia in patients with gastroesophageal reflux disease. Ann Surg 2001;234:627–32.

37. Patti MG, Arcerito M, Feo CV, et al. Barrett's esophagus: a surgical disease. J Gastrointest Surg 1999;3:397–403.

38. Oelschlager BK, Barreca M, Chang L, et al. Clinical and pathologic response of Barrett's esophagus to laparoscopic antireflux surgery. Ann Surg 2003;238: 458–64.

39. Bowers SP, Mattar SG, Smith CD, et al. Clinical and histologic follow-up after antireflux surgery for Barrett's esophagus. J Gastrointest Surg 2002;6:532–8.

40. Patti MG, Corvera CU, Glasgow RE, et al. A hospital's annual rate of esophagectomy influences the operative mortality rate. J Gastrointest Surg 1998;2:186–92.

41. Gasper WJ, Glidden DV, Way LW, et al. Has recognition of the relationship between mortality rates and hospital volume for major cancer surgery in California made a difference? A follow-up analysis of another decade. Ann Surg 2009; 250:472–83.

42. Ell C, May A, Pech O, et al. Curative endoscopic resection of early esophageal adenocarcinomas (Barrett's cancer). Gastrointest Endosc 2007;65:3–10.

43. Shaheen NJ, Sharma P, Overholt BF, et al. Radiofrequency ablation in Barrett's esophagus with dysplasia. N Engl J Med 2009;360:2277–88.

44. Weston AP, Sharma P, Topalovsky M, et al. Long-term follow-up of Barrett's high grade dysplasia. Am J Gastroenterol 2000;95:1888–93.
45. Reid BJ, Blount PL, Feng Z, et al. Optimizing endoscopic biopsy detection of early cancers in Barrett's high grade dysplasia. Am J Gastroenterol 2000;95: 3089–96.
46. Konda VJ, Ross AS, Ferguson MK, et al. Is the risk of concomitant invasive esophageal cancer in high-grade dysplasia in Barrett's Esophagus overestimated? Clin Gastroenterol Hepatol 2008;6:159–64.
47. Montgomery E, Bronner MP, Goldblum JR, et al. Reproducibility of the diagnosis of dysplasia in Barrett's esophagus: a reaffirmation. Hum Pathol 2001;32:368–78.
48. Penanthur A, Farkas A, Krasinskas AM, et al. Esophagectomy for T1 esophageal cancer: outcomes in 100 patients and implications for endoscopic therapy. Ann Thorac Surg 2009;87:1048–55.
49. Pech O, Beherens A, May A, et al. Long-term results and risk factor analysis for recurrence after curative endoscopic therapy in 349 patients with high-grade intraepithelial neoplasia and mucosal adenocarcinoma in Barrett's esophagus. Gut 2008;57:1200–6.
50. Badreddine RJ, Prasad GA, Wang KK, et al. Prevalence and predictors of recurrent neoplasia after ablation of Barrett's esophagus. Gastrointest Endosc 2010; 71:697–703.
51. Chang LL, Oelschalger BK, Quiroga E, et al. Long-term outcome of esophagectomy for high-grade dysplasia or cancer found during surveillance for Barrett's esophagus. J Gastrointest Surg 2006;10:341–6.

Endoscopic Interventions in Barrett's Esophagus: Do the Dollars Make Sense?

Jennifer Chennat, MD[a],*, Mark K. Ferguson, MD[b]

KEYWORDS

- Barrett's esophagus • Cost analysis • Cost-effectiveness
- Endoscopic ablation • Endoscopic therapy

Advances in the development of endoscopic therapies for Barrett's esophagus (BE) have resulted in the emergence of a variety of treatment options for this condition, particularly regarding management of early neoplasia. The published results of these modalities have demonstrated promising efficacy and safety. Long-term clinical data have been collected on some techniques but are still awaited on others. These surgery-sparing options have dramatically changed the treatment paradigm of BE and have potentially important implications for disease management and health care delivery from a cost perspective.

The major endoscopic treatment modalities used today include photodynamic therapy (PDT), endoscopic mucosal resection (EMR), multipolar electrocoagulation (MPEC), argon plasma coagulation, radiofrequency ablation (RFA), and cryotherapy. This article reviews the current literature on the cost analyses of these commonly used Barrett endoscopic interventions and summarizes the overall cost-effectiveness of these treatments as compared with surveillance or surgery. Understanding the issues that contribute to the economics of BE is critical for health care professionals, affected patients and their families, and those whose responsibilities require decision-making based on costs imposed on either patients or health care organizations.

NATURAL HISTORY OF BARRETT'S ESOPHAGUS AND COST IMPLICATIONS

The natural history of BE must be factored into cost evaluations of its various endoscopic interventions. Based on a simulation model confirmed by data from the US

The authors have nothing to disclose.
[a] Section of Gastroenterology, Department of Medicine, Center for Endoscopic Research and Therapeutics (CERT), The University of Chicago Medical Center, 5758 South Maryland Avenue, MC 9028, Chicago, IL 60637, USA
[b] Section of Thoracic Surgery, Department of Surgery, The University of Chicago Medical Center, 5841 South Maryland Avenue, MC 5035, Chicago, IL 60637, USA
* Corresponding author.
E-mail address: jchennat@medicine.bsd.uchicago.edu

Gastrointest Endoscopy Clin N Am 21 (2011) 145–153
doi:10.1016/j.giec.2010.09.004
1052-5157/11/$ – see front matter © 2011 Elsevier Inc. All rights reserved.

Surveillance, Epidemiology and End Results (SEER) cancer registry, an estimated prevalence for BE in the general population of 5.6% (5.49%–5.70%) accurately reflects reported incidence rates for esophageal adenocarcinoma (EAC).[1] The overall prevalence of BE in the setting of chronic reflux is as high as 10%.[2] Moreover, the annual risk of developing EAC in the setting of BE is 0.5% to 1.0%.[3–5] These general statistics influence clinical management decisions for varying degrees of BE neoplasia from endoscopic screening to surveillance to therapies. Although it is generally believed that EAC develops in the setting of BE through a progressive dysplastic sequence, the data regarding rates of cancer progression for varying degrees of dysplasia are inherently flawed due to issues, such as spontaneous regression, sampling error, interobserver histologic assessment variability, and overestimation of effect in observational studies.[6,7] Despite these limitations, the presence and extent of dysplasia within the BE segment provides the ability to risk-stratify patients based on its severity, which has implications on deciding whether or not to subject a patient to a medical intervention.

Screening for BE and surveillance for dysplasia and cancer remain controversial issues. Current guidelines advise that the highest yields for diagnosing the condition are in patients ages greater than 50 years, patients who are white, and patients who have long-standing heartburn. In addition, despite debates about cost-benefit profiles and cost-effectiveness, society guidelines continue to support the use of surveillance programs for BE patients both with and without dysplasia at varying frequency intervals.[8–11]

Even the mere diagnosis of BE without dysplasia can have profound effects on patients' life insurance premiums due to insurers' concerns about abbreviated life expectancy of policy holders due to an increased risk of developing EAC. In a survey study of 20 US-based life insurance companies (10 in southern California and 10 in North Carolina), investigators found that, for a base case, an otherwise healthy 43-year-old man with no BE, the yearly preferred life insurance averaged $1255. For the same-aged individual with BE as a pre-existing condition, the mean cost of policies offered was $2731 (P<.001). In the case of a 36-year-old woman with no documented medical conditions, the rate ranged from $472 to $551. With the addition of a BE diagnosis, the mean rate rose by 177%, to $1434, with a range of $1144 to $1896.[12] Thus, endoscopic treatments aimed at eradication of BE must also study the issues surrounding overall risk reduction for EAC and recurrence of BE in the post-ablation esophagus. This is paramount, because these factors have bearing on health care and insurance costs, and potential for patient labeling in society due to the rationale that mere eradication of BE may only temporarily eliminate the BE disease state and may not confer long-term protection against disease-related complications.

ECONOMICS OF BARRETT'S ESOPHAGUS ENDOSCOPIC THERAPIES

The majority of cost-effectiveness analyses pertaining to BE have focused on screening or surveillance programs. With the emergence of endoscopic therapies demonstrating acceptable safety and efficacy profiles, recent data have emerged comparing costs related to these modalities to either surveillance or surgery alternatives. Initial cost studies focused on endoscopic ablation with PDT, which was the first nonsurgical modality demonstrated to have durable and efficacious results.

To delineate the best management strategy for high-grade dysplasia (HGD), researchers have used decision analytic modeling to systematically assess various clinical options. In one study, the four main arms included no preventative strategy, elective esophagectomy, endoscopic ablation (PDT in this study), and surveillance endoscopy for a base case healthy 50-year-old white man with an initial diagnosis of BE with HGD. The most effective strategy was endoscopic ablation, yielding 15.5 discounted quality-adjusted life years (QALYs) compared with 15.0 for surveillance endoscopy and 14.9 for surgery. The most inexpensive option, as expected, was having no preventative strategy. This choice had an average cost per QALY of $54. It resulted, however, in high rates of cancer. Endoscopic surveillance was less expensive and more effective than esophagectomy. Additionally, through a phenomenon called extended dominance, although the total costs of ablation were greater than surveillance, an additional life year was less expensive to purchase through ablation than surveillance. The change in the ICER moving from no therapy to ablation was a reasonable $25,621 per QALY. Through sensitivity analyses, researchers found that when yearly rates of progression from HGD to cancer were greater than 30%, esophagectomy became the most cost-effective strategy.[2] These findings helped set the stage for the financial justifications for ablative technology use in the setting of BE with HGD.

Another group also studied the most cost-effective strategy to manage BE HGD and any residual disease present after endoscopic treatment. Four strategies were evaluated: esophagectomy, endoscopic surveillance, PDT followed by esophagectomy for residual HGD, and PDT followed by endoscopic surveillance for residual HGD. They found that esophagectomy cost $24,045, with life expectancy of 11.82 QALY. PDT followed by endoscopic surveillance for residual HGD was the most effective strategy, with a life expectancy of 12.31 QALY. It also incurred the greatest lifetime cost ($47,310), however, resulting in an incremental cost-effectiveness of $47,410 per QALY.[13]

As the efficacy of various ablative technologies began to gain recognition during the first decade of the twenty-first century, a landmark cost-utility analysis was published to help guide future cost assessment studies. In a decision analytic model created to examine a BE patient population with a mean age of 50 years, separate subanalyses were conducted for patients with no dysplasia, low-grade dysplasia (LGD), or HGD. The management strategies compared were endoscopic surveillance, endoscopic surveillance with ablation for incident dysplasia, immediate ablation followed by endoscopic surveillance in all patients or limited to patients in whom metaplasia persisted, and esophagectomy. The ablation modalities included in the model were RFA, APC, MPEC, and PDT.[14]

The primary outcome of the study was measurement of the incremental cost per QALY between the analyzed management strategies, also known as the incremental cost-effectiveness ratio (ICER). This ratio is defined as the cost difference when moving from a less expensive but less effective strategy, to a more expensive but more effective strategy, divided by the change in QALYs between these two strategies. The study showed that endoscopic ablation for HGD could increase life expectancy of patients by 3 quality-adjusted years at an incremental cost of less than $6000 compared with no intervention. In the base case analysis of 50-year-old patients with BE and HGD, endoscopic ablation with PDT, RFA, or APC with postablation endoscopic surveillance was calculated to extend life by 3.2 QALYs compared with performing no surveillance. MPEC did not have any data reported for use in BE with HGD. APC and RFA demonstrated cost increases of $19,000 to $20,000 per person, and PDT costs were $30,000 greater than no surveillance. Comparing RFA with performing no surveillance demonstrated an acceptable ICER of $5839 per QALY gained. The ICER calculated with PDT, however, required an overwhelming $32 million per QALY gained.[14]

Patients with LGD or no dysplasia could also be optimally managed with ablation, but it was expensive to continue surveillance after eradication of metaplasia. Ablation was preferred to surveillance if ablation permanently eradicated greater than 28% of LGD or 40% of nondysplastic metaplasia. The investigators concluded that endoscopic ablation could be the preferred strategy for managing patients with BE and HGD. The unknown long-term effectiveness of ablation for BE, however, with either LGD or no dysplasia influenced the overall cost-effectiveness of this approach for these disease states in an unfavorable manner.[14]

With respect to management of stage 0 or 1 esophageal cancer (adenocarcinoma or squamous cell cancer), a systematic review of the SEER database has shown the long-term survival of endoscopic resection with or without ablation using PDT or thermal therapy is comparable with that of surgery.[15] Concerning BE-related early cancer (T1 with mucosal or minimal submucosal infiltration), a decision tree model compared EMR of the cancerous lesion with RFA of the remaining Barrett segment to esophagectomy. During the 5-year interval of the study, endoscopic therapy cost $17,000. and yielded 4.88 QALYs, compared with $28,000 and 4.59, respectively, for esophagectomy. The overall outcome was not changed by varying the recurrence rates of cancer or BE metaplasia after endoscopic therapy. Even under the most optimal circumstances favoring esophagectomy, such as 2% operative mortality rate, no reduced quality of life (QOL) after esophagectomy, and a low 5-year survival rate after recurrence associated with endoscopic ablation, the risk of positive lymph nodes still needed to exceed 25% before esophagectomy became the preferred treatment option.[16] The threshold for risk of lymph node invasion in the setting of submucosal invasion for which it is significant enough to warrant the greater invasiveness and cost involved with esophagectomy over endoscopic resection remains to be clearly defined.

The extent of reduction of EAC after BE ablation therapy also deserves more scrutiny, because this may have bearing on long-term and overall costs. In a pooled analysis of natural history of BE and ablation of BE articles, the rates of cancer in patients undergoing ablation and from the natural history were calculated. Ablation was associated with a reduction in cancer incidence with the greatest benefit observed in the BE HGD subgroup, although these findings may have been limited by the heterogenous nature of the included studies.[17]

Increasing attention has been given to endoscopic ablation of LGD and nondysplastic BE due to concerns about potential neoplastic progression. A recent study reported that approximately 85% of 147 patients who carried the diagnosis of LGD before expert pathology review actually had no dysplasia. For patients who had a consensus diagnosis of LGD, the cumulative risk of progression to HGD or cancer was 85% in 109.1 months as compared with 4.6% in 107.4 months for patients down-staged to nondysplastic BE ($P<.0001$) on the basis of expert review. Thus, BE with LGD is an overdiagnosed entity with an underestimated neoplastic potential.[18] In addition to the presence of LGD, the extent of LGD is a significant risk factor for the development of esophageal adenocarcinoma. Even though the presence of HGD is associated with a significantly greater relative risk for development of cancer, the extent of HGD is not an independent risk factor for progression to cancer.[19]

With these issues in mind, endoscopic ablation has been proposed for LGD and nondysplastic BE. In a Markov model, three competing strategies were evaluated in a hypothetical 50-year-old cohort with nondysplastic BE, allowing for the natural history to be modeled for various health and disease states associated with a different set of utilities (**Fig. 1**). These three strategies were (1) no surveillance, (2) surveillance, and (3) endoscopic ablation. The model was biased against ablation with a conservative estimate of complete response and continued standard surveillance even after complete ablation. All potential complications were considered, and an incomplete

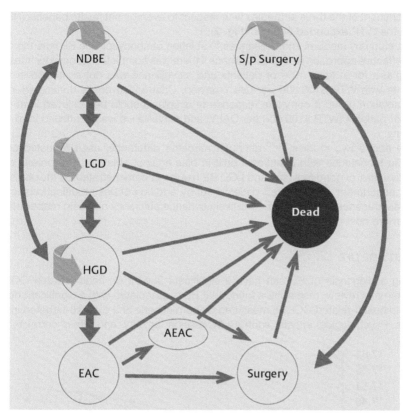

Fig. 1. Markov model showing the natural history of BE patients with various health and disease states, associated with different sets of utilities. A single arrow indicates transition from one state to another. Double arrows indicate transitions allowed in both directions in the model. Semicircle arrows represent states in which a patient can remain indefinitely. AEAC, advanced esophageal adenocarcinoma; NDBE, nondysplastic BE; S/p, status post. (*From* Das A, Wells C, Kim HJ, et al. An economic analysis of endoscopic ablative therapy for management of nondysplastic Barrett's esophagus. Endoscopy 2009;41:400–8; with permission.)

histologic response after ablation was presumed to have the same neoplastic risk of progression as a case of untreated BE. Patients in the surveillance arm who demonstrated nondysplastic BE would undergo repeat endoscopy every 3 years. Those who demonstrated LGD would have surveillance endoscopy performed every 1 year until no dysplasia was detected. Those with focal HGD would have repeat EGD and biopsy by endoscopic surveillance every 3 months. All patients with persistent, diffuse or multifocal HGD and cancers were considered for surgical resection. Endoscopic surveillance was allowed up to the age of 80 years. The model was constructed to allow for misdiagnosis of histologic specimens, based on available published false-positive and false-negative rates. The ablative strategy yielded the highest QALYs and was more cost-effective than surveillance. The incremental cost to gain an extra QALY with the strategy of ablation was $48,626 compared with the endoscopic surveillance strategy. By current standard of cost-effective medical interventions, a strategy with an incremental cost of $50,000 or less per QALY gained is deemed acceptable in terms of society's willingness to pay (WTP). Endoscopic ablation was the dominant of the three strategies with respect to average net health benefits (NHBs) when the WTP exceeded $60,000 (**Fig. 2**).[20]

In a study by Inadomi and colleagues,[14] ablation of nondysplastic BE was the most cost-effective approach versus surveillance if there was complete response for intestinal metaplasia for at least 40% of patients and surveillance was not continued in such patients with WTP $100,000 per QALY gained. Cost-effectiveness dominated in the LGD ablation group if complete response of dysplasia could be achieved in at least 28% of patients (WTP $100,000 per QALY) and surveillance was continued in all LGD patients.

The above two studies,[14,20] although modeled differently, used robust decision analytic techniques with intentional built-in bias against ablation. Reasonable cost-effectiveness of nondysplastic and LGD BE has been demonstrated by these results. Thus, enrichment of a targeted patient pool by addition of risk stratification factors, such as presence of biomarkers, will likely enhance efficiency and help make ablation even more cost effective.[21]

QUALITY OF LIFE

Having a diagnosis of BE can have a significant impact on health-related QOL. In a systematic review, researchers found that BE is associated with a significant decrement in health-related QOL as measured by both generic and disease-targeted instruments. Psychological effects, such as depression, anxiety, and stress correlate with

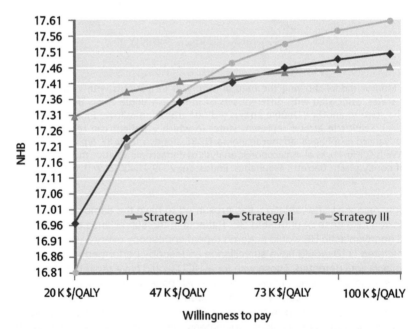

Fig. 2. The Y axis represents the average NHBs yielded under each of the three strategies and is plotted against the X axis, WTP. Endoscopic surveillance does not yield incremental NHB compared with the no preventative intervention strategy until the WTP exceeds approximately $75,000. Endoscopic ablation yields the highest NHB and is the dominant of all three strategies, at a WTP of approximately $60,000 or higher. (*From* Das A, Wells C, Kim HJ, et al. An economic analysis of endoscopic ablative therapy for management of nondysplastic Barrett's esophagus. Endoscopy 2009;41:400–8; with permission.)

knowledge of disease potential which may be related to their increased risk of cancer. A diagnosis of BE also leads to increased health care use and spending when compared with patients with gastroesophageal reflux disease or the general population.[22,23]

The QOL comparisons between esophagectomy and endoscopic therapies are still not mature. The 36-Item Short Form Health Survey and the Gastrointestinal Quality of Life Index questionnaire were sent to all patients who underwent either esophagectomy or endoscopic therapy for early neoplasia in a single-center study. Surveys were sent to 77 patients and were completed by 50% of the esophagectomy and 57% of the endoscopically treated patients. In age-matched controls, esophagectomy and endoscopic treatment for early Barrett neoplasia had similar impact on QOL 1 year or more after intervention. Younger patients undergoing surgery seemed to have a greater negative QOL impact compared with endoscopic therapy.[24]

As endoscopic interventions continue to report efficacy and safety data, they will increasingly be used in mainstream clinical practice and larger-scale outcomes can be accrued. One of the goals of studies of endoscopic BE therapies should include the use of sophisticated and specific QOL measures to determine the impact these therapies have compared with control cohorts, such as surveillance or surgical patients. This aspect of health care delivery will be integral to eventual widespread adoption or rejection of endoscopic therapies for BE in all its stages by physicians and their patients.

SUMMARY

The widespread clinical incorporation of various endoscopic interventions for BE carries significant potential to alter the natural history of the disease while sparing patients expensive surgical or indefinite surveillance alternatives. Although promising data are emerging on efficacy and safety profiles of these modalities, the durability of this data needs to be confirmed over time. Based on current data, BE with HGD is most cost-effectively treated by RFA. EMR is cost preferred to esophagectomy for early BE cancer, although more definitive modeled comparisons of cost-effectiveness between these two strategies for management of early cancer are still needed. Endoscopic ablation of BE with LGD or no dysplasia requires additional outcomes data before generalized recommendations can be made.

More comprehensive comparative analyses of direct health care costs and QOL assessments are two research frontiers that require enhanced systematic data collection to substantiate the use of these endoscopic modalities for a variety of indications in the setting of BE. Areas of future investigative focus should also include the cost implications of complete response to endoscopic therapy, determination of the role of surveillance in the postablative esophagus, and assessment of indirect costs to patients and family members. Only then will an accurate perspective be gained on the issue of whether or not these endoscopic intervention dollars are ultimately cost saving for society overall.

REFERENCES

1. Hayeck TJ, Kong CY, Spechler SJ, et al. The prevalence of Barrett's esophagus in the US: estimates from a simulation model confirmed by SEER data. Dis Esophagus 2010;23(6):451–7.
2. Shaheen NJ, Inadomi JM, Overholt BF, et al. What is the best management strategy for high grade dysplasia in Barrett's oesophagus? A cost effectiveness analysis. Gut 2004;53:1736–44.

3. Thomas T, Abrams KR, De Caestecker JS, et al. Meta analysis: cancer risk in Barrett's oesophagus. Aliment Pharmacol Ther 2007;26:1465–77.
4. Spechler SJ. The natural history of dysplasia and cancer in esophagitis and Barrett esophagus. J Clin Gastroenterol 2003;36:S2–8.
5. Shaheen NJ, Crosby MA, Bozymski EM, et al. Is there publication bias in the reporting of cancer risk in Barrett's esophagus? Gastroenterology 2000;119: 333–8.
6. Spechler SJ. Dysplasia in Barrett's esophagus: limitations of current management strategies. Am J Gastroenterol 2005;100:927–35.
7. Shaheen NJ, Spechler SJ. Total endoscopic eradication of Barrett's esophagus: study methodology, candidate selection, and clinical outcomes. Endoscopy 2008;40:994–9.
8. Wang KK, Wongkeesong M, Buttar NS. American gastroenterological association technical review on the role of the gastroenterologist in the management of esophageal carcinoma. Gastroenterology 2005;128:1471–505.
9. Wang KK, Wongkeesong M, Buttar NS. American Gastroenterological Association medical position statement: role of the gastroenterologist in the management of esophageal carcinoma. Gastroenterology 2005;128:1468–70.
10. SSAT patient care guidelines. Management of Barrett's esophagus. J Gastrointest Surg 2007;11:1213–5.
11. Wang KK, Sampliner RE. Updated guidelines 2008 for the diagnosis, surveillance and therapy of Barrett's esophagus. Am J Gastroenterol 2008;103:788–97.
12. Shaheen NJ, Dulai GS, Ascher B, et al. Effect of a new diagnosis of Barrett's esophagus on insurance status. Am J Gastroenterol 2005;100:577–80.
13. Vij R, Triadafilopoulos G, Owens DK, et al. Cost-effectiveness of photodynamic therapy for high-grade dysplasia in Barrett's esophagus. Gastrointest Endosc 2004;60:739–56.
14. Inadomi JM, Somsouk M, Madanick RD, et al. A cost-utility analysis of ablative therapy for Barrett's esophagus. Gastroenterology 2009;136:2101–14, e1–6.
15. Das A, Singh V, Fleischer DE, et al. A comparison of endoscopic treatment and surgery in early esophageal cancer: an analysis of surveillance epidemiology and end results data. Am J Gastroenterol 2008;103:1340–5.
16. Pohl H, Sonnenberg A, Strobel S, et al. Endoscopic versus surgical therapy for early cancer in Barrett's esophagus: a decision analysis. Gastrointest Endosc 2009;70:623–31.
17. Wani S, Puli SR, Shaheen NJ, et al. Esophageal adenocarcinoma in Barrett's esophagus after endoscopic ablative therapy: a meta-analysis and systematic review. Am J Gastroenterol 2009;104:502–13.
18. Curvers WL, Ten Kate FJ, Krishnadath KK, et al. Low-grade dysplasia in Barrett's esophagus: overdiagnosed and underestimated. Am J Gastroenterol 2010; 105(7):1523–30.
19. Srivastava A, Hornick JL, Li X, et al. Extent of low-grade dysplasia is a risk factor for the development of esophageal adenocarcinoma in Barrett's esophagus. Am J Gastroenterol 2007;102:483–94.
20. Das A, Wells C, Kim HJ, et al. An economic analysis of endoscopic ablative therapy for management of nondysplastic Barrett's esophagus. Endoscopy 2009;41:400–8.
21. Fleischer DE, Odze R, Overholt BF, et al. The case for endoscopic treatment of non-dysplastic and low-grade dysplastic Barrett's esophagus. Dig Dis Sci 2010;55:1918–31.

22. Crockett SD, Lippmann QK, Dellon ES, et al. Health-related quality of life in patients with Barrett's esophagus: a systematic review. Clin Gastroenterol Hepatol 2009;7:613–23.
23. Gerson LB, Ullah N, Hastie T, et al. Does cancer risk affect health-related quality of life in patients with Barrett's esophagus? Gastrointest Endosc 2007;65:16–25.
24. Schembre D, Arai A, Levy S, et al. Quality of life after esophagectomy and endoscopic therapy for Barrett's esophagus with dysplasia. Dis Esophagus 2010; 23(6):458–64.

Chemoprevention in Barrett's Esophagus: A Pill a Day?

Janusz A. Jankowski, MSc(Oxon), MD(Dund), PhD(Lond), FRCP(Lond)[a,b,c,*],
Patricia A. Hooper, MBChB(Leics), BSc(Leics)[a]

KEYWORDS

- Barrett's esophagus • Esophageal adenocarcinoma
- Chemoprevention • Aspirin

Esophageal cancer is continuing to increase at a fast rate with a 40-fold increase in prevalence over the past 40 years. This rise is mainly due to the ongoing increase in incidence of esophageal adenocarcinoma (EAC), the predominant histologic type in the United States and the United Kingdom.[1] Despite improvements in surgical and oncologic treatment, prognosis of those diagnosed with EAC remains poor, with an overall 5-year survival of less than 15%. The main risk factor for EAC is the premalignant condition of Barrett's esophagus (BE). BE is common, affecting 10% to 15% of those who undergo upper gastrointestinal endoscopy for reflux symptoms. Its incidence is rising.[2] BE is also underdiagnosed; with an autopsy study finding for every known case, 20 remain undiagnosed.[3]

Progression from BE to EAC occurs at a rate of 0.5% to 1% per patient year of follow-up[4,5] and patients have a 30- to 125-times increased risk of developing EAC compared with the general population. Those most at risk include white men of increasing age; smokers; those with frequent, severe reflux of long duration; and those with low fruit and vegetable intake with a raised body mass index (BMI). Helicobacter cagA strain is thought to be protective. Incidence of EAC is highest in the United Kingdom (5.8 to 8.7 per 100,000), followed by Australia (4.8 per 100,000), Netherlands (4.4 per 100,000), and the United States (3.7 per 100,000).[6] The progression from Barrett to adenocarcinoma occurs via a multistep process through squamous epithelium to columnar-lined epithelium, specialized intestinal metaplasia to low-grade dysplasia (LGD), high-grade dysplasia (HGD), and adenocarcinoma with later invasion and metastasis. This process is thought to develop slowly over several years, which

Janusz A. Jankowski is a consultant to Astrazeneca (Macclesfield, UK).

[a] Digestive Diseases Centre, Leicester Royal Infirmary, Infirmary Square, Leicester, LE1 5WW, UK
[b] Department of Clinical Pharmacology, University of Oxford, Oxford, OX3 7DQ, UK
[c] Centre for Digestive Diseases, Queen Mary University of London, London, E1 2AT, UK
* Corresponding author. Digestive Diseases Centre, Leicester Royal Infirmary, Infirmary Square, Leicester, LE1 5WW, UK.
E-mail address: j.a.jankowski@qmul.ac.uk

Gastrointest Endoscopy Clin N Am 21 (2011) 155–170
doi:10.1016/j.giec.2010.09.005
1052-5157/11/$ – see front matter © 2011 Elsevier Inc. All rights reserved.

giendo.theclinics.com

lends BE as a perfect model with which to study chemoprevention. Median time to diagnosis of columnar-lined esophagus from start of symptoms was 2.6 years, to intestinal metaplasia 5.0 years, and to LGD 30 years in a large (1082 patients), multi-center cohort study[7]; 10% had HGD at 9.6 years and 10% EAC at 13.8 years in the same cohort. The aim of chemoprevention is to prevent or slow the progression along the metaplastic-dysplastic carcinoma spectrum to allow cancers to be prevented or picked up at an earlier stage to allow more effective treatment by earlier intervention.

PARADIGM OF CHEMOPREVENTION

EAC is an aggressive disease with poor prognosis, making chemoprevention a desirable prospect. The few treatment options are associated with high mortality and morbidity. Despite an increased understanding of the progression of the disease and advances in surgical techniques, mortality from this condition has changed little. The alternative strategies to preventing or reducing mortality from Barrett associated EAC are not without their controversies. These include screening, surveillance to pick up EAC before symptomatic presentation, lifestyle modifications, treatment of HGD, and identification of biomarkers that predispose individuals to a higher risk of developing EAC (Fig. 1). Surveillance is proposed as cost effective when the incidence of cancer is at least 0.5% to 1%. Less than this is not cost effective; therefore, the rate of malignant transformation is pivotal. If EAC is picked up at a stage when it is confined to the esophagus, there is a 70% 5-year survival. Challenges facing surveillance include low adherence to guidelines and considerable inter- and intraobserver

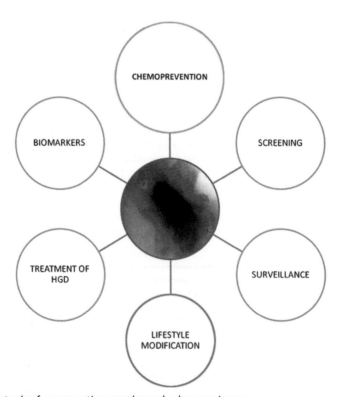

Fig. 1. Strategies for preventing esophageal adenocarcinoma.

variations between pathologists on the degree of dysplasia present.[8] The authors hope to see downstaging of EAC and not just a longer lead time. This has to be balanced against the morbidity and mortality associated with surveillance. It has been proposed that surveillance combined with chemoprevention is a cost-effective way of preventing EAC. Smoking and raised BMI are associated with an increased risk of developing EAC. Patients with a raised BMI are also more likely to develop BE.

However, none of these are yet adequately validated for clinical use. Identifying those patients most at risk of developing cancer means chemoprevention can be effectively tailored toward those most at need to optimize the risk-benefit ratio and minimize risk of side-effects of chemoprevention to those at lower risk.[9] Biomarkers predicting malignant potential are currently being studied. These include p16, p53, cyclin D1, aneuploidy, tetraploidy, E-cadherin, tumor necrosis factor a (TNF-a), b-catenin, c-Myc, cyclooxygenase 2 (COX-2), and prostaglandin E2 (PGE2).

A good chemoprevention agent needs to be effective at reducing EAC, with an acceptable side-effect profile. It also needs to be cost effective and acceptable to patients taking it. EAC has a low incidence even in patients with BE; therefore, chemoprevention trials need large numbers of patients with long follow-up and a safe medication. The cost-effectiveness of screening and chemoprevention relies on how effective the medication is at preventing progression to cancer. Chemoprevention is more cost effective in high-risk groups, such as those with HGD, even in higher-cost or less-effective interventions.[10] Approaches to chemoprevention include targeting those at high risk or using a safe medication with other recognized health benefits.[11] Compliance is a major issue with chemoprevention. Patients generally feel well. Compliance of taking aspirin (100 mg) on alternate days was 75% at 5 years and 67% at 10 years. A study of 39,876 women showed no protective benefit of aspirin in preventing any cancers. If study subjects fall short of good compliance, the general population may do even less well.[12] A chemopreventive agent that was safe, cheap, effective, and acceptable would have great impact on not only on cancer reduction but also on health economics.

POSSIBLE AGENTS

There are no agents licensed currently for chemoprevention in BE. There have been many agents suggested as having a chemopreventive effect (**Fig. 2**). The medications gaining the most interest have been nonsteroidal anti-inflammatory drugs (NSAIDs), including COX-2 inhibitors and aspirin, and proton pump inhibitors (PPIs). Others that have been suggested include statins, green tea, antioxidants, vitamins A and E, curcumin, telomerase inhibitors, folic acid, berries, ornithine decarboxylase, matrix metalloproteinase inhibitors, and anti–vascular endothelial growth factor (VEGF) monoclonal antibodies. The role and research of some of these agents are discussed, with particular focus on NSAIDs and PPIs.

Food Groups

A large prospective cohort study followed 490,802 people for 2,193,751 person years of follow-up. High fruit and vegetable intake was found to reduce the risk of developing esophageal squamous cell carcinoma (hazard ratio [HR] 0.78; 95% CI, [0.57–0.93] but not EAC HR 0.98 [0.9–1.08]), with stronger protective relationship for fruit when analyzed further. There was an inverse relationship between intake of Chenopodiaceae (spinach) and risk of developing EAC (HR 0.66; 95% CI, [0.46–0.95]), with a nonsignificant trend toward cruciferae being protective, suggesting green vegetables containing nutrients, such as isothiocyanates, may be protective.[13] A further,

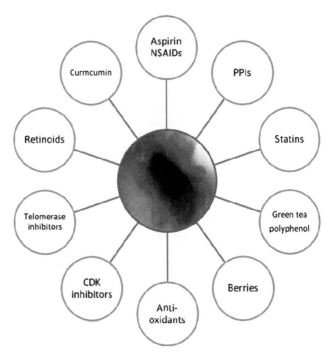

Fig. 2. Possible agents for chemoprevention in Barrett's esophagus.

retrospective population-based case-control study was performed by Chen and colleagues.[14] They interviewed 124 EAC patients, 124 distal gastric cancer patients, and 449 controls (or their proxy) about their food intake in the years before diagnosis. They found those with highest intake of vitamin A, β-cryptoxanthin, riboflavin, folate, zinc, fiber, protein, and carbohydrates were associated with a 40% to 50% lower incidence of EAC than those consuming the lowest amounts and found increased risk with those found consuming the most fat. The study was potentially limited by the risk of recall bias. Folate and riboflavin (necessary for DNA metabolism) deficiencies also interfere with DNA repair and methylation.

Antioxidants

Low manganese superoxide dismutase (MnSOD) levels are associated with higher rates of BE and EAC. Supplementation of MnSOD in animal models has been shown to reduce oxidative stress DNA injury and has been proposed for preventing malignant transformation.[15]

Cyclin-Dependent Kinase Inhibitors

Flavopiridol (cyclin-dependent kinase inhibitor) reduced the prevalence of BE and EAC in p27-deficient mice. Down-regulation of cyclin D1 occurred. Limitations of use as a chemopreventive agent include intravenous administration and side-effects, such as diarrhea, asthenia, neutropenia, and clotting problems.[16]

Retinoic Acid

Retinoids have been trialed as a chemopreventive agent; however, the trial was halted due to side-effect of esophaeal ulceration. Dietary deficiency of β-carotene (vitamin A provitamin) is associated with increased risk of EAC in epidemiologic studies. All-*trans* retinoic acid has been shown to induce apoptosis and increases p53 expression in a metaplastic Barrett cell line. The development of less toxic retinoids may play a future role in chemoprevention.[17]

Telomerase Inhibitors

Telomerase activity has been shown elevated in Barrett adenocarcinoma cell lines. It is thought that Barrett EAC stimulated telomerase, leading to unchecked proliferation. Use of 2,6-bis[3-(N-piperidino)propionamido]anthracene-9,10-dione (PPA), a G-complex intercalating telomerase inhibitor, led to growth arrest, reduced colony number and increased apoptosis and reduction in telomerase activity, raising the possibility of use in chemoprevention.[18]

Lyophilized Black Raspberries

Lyophilized black raspberries have been shown in animal models to reduce cancer development in gastrointestinal tract cancers, and research in vitro has supported this. Kresty and colleagues[19] performed a trial of the use of lyophilized black raspberries daily for 6 months in patients with BE. They measured urinary markers of oxidative stress in these patients and found a marked reduction. Significant weight gain was observed during the study postulated as due to extra calories consumed from the raspberries.

Polyphenols

Polyphenols are found in green tea and berries, among other products. Green tea consumption in Asian studies is linked to a lower rate of several cancers, including colorectal cancer. Polyphenols have been shown to exert a chemopreventive effect in carcinogenic cell line studies. Resveratol is found in grape skin and red wine. It is thought to exert an antioxidant effect. In animal studies, a reduction of intestinal metaplasia and cancer was found, but this did not reach statistical significance.[20]

Proton Pump Inhibitors

In a Minnesota population, 19.8% reported at least weekly reflux symptoms, and prevalence of heartburn was 42%.[21] The most intuitive agents for chemoprevention of EAC seem to be PPIs. These are used to improve gastroesophageal reflux disease symptoms and induce mucosal healing in erosive reflux esophagitis that makes diagnosis of Barrett and dysplasia more difficult. Use of PPIs since their release 20 years ago has rocketed, but the rate of EAC has not been reduced; it has increased exponentially during this time. Those patients with regular heartburn (once a week) had 7.7% increased risk of developing EAC. The longest duration of gastroesophageal reflux (more than 20 years) and more severe symptoms were associated with a 43.3 odds ratio (OR) of developing EAC.[22] The Factors Influencing the Barrett's Adenocarcinoma Relationship (FINBAR) study found patients with BE 18 times more likely (and those with EAC 3 times more likely) than controls to have severe reflux and reflux of longer duration.[23] Because reflux is associated with increased risk of EAC, it seems logical that by treating reflux the risk of developing cancer also is reduced. It has been shown that even when rendered asymptomatic from gastroesophageal reflux with lansoprazole (15–30 mg), 40% of patients with BE had incomplete acid suppression as judged by 24-hour pH studies. Therefore, if the aim of treatment is effective acid suppression, 24-hour pH studies may be necessary to titrate doses.[24] Barrett mucosa is less sensitive than squamous epithelium. This study demonstrates symptoms guiding reflux treatment are not reliable.

An Australian study of 350 patients with BE, with a mean follow-up of 4.7 years, found use of PPIs reduced progression to LGD and HGD. The investigators found that patients who used PPI therapy had a mean time to diagnosis of LGD of 14.1 years (95% CI, 13.1–15.0); 19% developed LGD during the study, in contrast to those who did not start a PPI on enrollment in a mean time to diagnosis of 8.8 years. Within 3.2 years of enrollment, 50% developed LGD.[25] A delay of 2 years in commencing PPI therapy led to 5.6-times increased risk of LGD, compared with those starting a PPI within a year of commencing surveillance, and to 20.9-times increased risk (2.8–158) of progressing to HGD or EAC compared with those whose PPI therapy was not delayed. A Veterans Affairs study found PPI use reduced the risk of development of EAC or HGD by 61%.[26] Lao-Sireix and colleagues[27] showed that effective acid suppression reduced proliferation in BE but had no effect on expression of COX-2, c-Myc, or apoptosis. Continuous acid suppression is desirable because pulsed therapy has been shown to induce proliferation and lead to dysplasia. Continuous acid suppression leads to differentiation and less risk of dysplasia.[28] PPI use is known to increase gastrin levels and hypergastrinemia has been associated with increased COX-2 expression.

ASPIRIN AND NSAIDS

Optimism for the use of aspirin and NSAIDs in chemoprevention against EAC comes from drawing a parallel with another gastrointestinal premalignant condition, colonic adenomatous polyps, where aspirin has been associated with reduced colorectal carcinoma development. Aspirin is also commonly used in primary and secondary prevention in cardiovascular disease (COV), a condition which occurs in excess and causes early mortality in patients with BE.[29] This could be due to shared risk factors (male gender, older age, smoking, poor lifestyle, reduced fresh fruit and vegetable intake, and raised BMI and adiposity) or due to shared genetic factors.

COX-2 is important in the development of many cancers. It reduces differentiation, increases proliferation, reduces cell adhesion, blocks apoptosis, and encourages angiogenesis, invasion, and later metastasis. COX-2 also increases cancer cell resistance to the immune response. The expression of COX-2 is increased with patients with BE, LGD, HGD, and EAC, although this is variable.[30] NSAIDs, including COX-2 inhibitors and aspirin, have been shown in in vitro and animal studies to reduce the development of EAC in Barrett cell lines. In animal studies, Buttar and colleagues[31] assessed the response of 16 weeks of treatment with MF-tricyclic (selective COX-2 inhibitor) and sulindac (nonselective COX-2 inhibitor) on rat models. They found that both significantly reduced the relative risk of esophageal cancer by 55% and 79%, respectively, and also reduced inflammation and COX-2 expression. They postulated that this supports the possible role of chemoprevention for COX-2 inhibitors in BE in preventing EAC. The same group also demonstrated that the in vitro selective COX-2 inhibitor, NS-398, decreased cell proliferation of Barrett cell lines by 55% (95% CI, 47.1–63.8) and reduced COX-2 activity.[32] Celecoxib has been shown to reduce incidence of esophagitis and columnar-lined epithelium in rat models. It was shown to increase apoptosis and decrease PGE2 levels.[33]

A prospective study of 350 patients with BE reported a substantially lower incidence of EAC in those patients who currently (6.6%) and previously (9.7%) used NSAIDs than those who had never taken it (14.3%).[34] Protective effect seemed to last through 30 months of follow-up but risk over time returned to baseline levels by 3 years. They also found a reduction in aneuploidy and tetraploidy. This study included a subgroup of patients with HGD. Those who used aspirin or NSAIDs had a lower rate of malignant transformation, indicating a role for chemoprevention even at an advanced stage.[34]

Selective COX-2 inhibitors were evaluated during the recent Chemoprevention for Barrett's Esophagus Trial, a phase IIb multicenter placebo trial, which recruited 100 patients who had confirmed BE with LGD and HGD. They randomized patients to receive BD celecoxib (200 mg twice a day) or placebo. They found no statistically significant difference in change in dysplasia from baseline with treatment with celecoxib. In the LGD group, change in the proportion of biopsies with dysplasia or cancer from baseline with celecoxib was –0.09 and with placebo –0.07 ($P = .64$); in the HGD group, treatment with celecoxib change was 0.12 and with placebo 0.02 ($P = .88$). They found no significant difference in the surface area of Barrett, prostaglandin levels, COX-1 and -2 mRNA, p16 methylation, adenomatous polyposis coli, or E-cadherin levels. Limitations highlighted included conservative dosing, inter- and intraobserver variations in dysplasia reporting, and natural regression of LGD or HGD.[35] Further analysis controlling baseline characteristics showed a reduction in the total Barrett surface area at 1 year.[36] In a separate study, celecoxib (200 mg twice daily for 28 days) reduced COX-2 expression by 20% and 44% in two separate biopsy sites in a patient with BE.[37] The main limitation to the use of COX-2 inhibitors is the increased cardiovascular risk profile. Rofecoxib showed promising results as a chemopreventive agent, with dosing of 25 mg daily for 10 days showing a 77% reduction in COX-2 expression, proliferation, and PGE2 release, contributing toward evidence for COX-2 inhibitors in chemoprevention; however, the cardiovascular risk profile has limited its use in this respect.[38]

Aspirin—A Leading Contender?

Aspirin possesses several key benefits to making it a leading contender for chemoprevention against EAC (**Table 1**). Aspirin is effective at reducing the risk of BE undergoing malignant progression to EAC. This has been supported by several case-control and cohort studies. It is widely used in primary and secondary prevention of ischemic events in those at high risk. A systematic review demonstrated a protective role for aspirin and NSAIDs in reducing EAC (OR 0.57; 95% CI, 0.67–0.99), when analyzed by medication type, aspirin was protective (OR 0.5; 95% CI, 0.38–0.66), whereas NSAIDs were borderline statistically significant (OR 0.75; 95% CI, 0.54–1.0). Greater protection was associated with more frequent aspirin use. This was true for both histologic types oesophageal squamous carcinoma and oesophageal adenocarcinoma.[39] A meta-analysis of 34 case-control and 13 cohort studies found a relative risk of developing EAC of 0.51 (95% CI, 0.38–0.69) when taking aspirin

Table 1 Beneficial properties of aspirin in chemoprevention	
Feature	**Aspirin**
Cheap	£3.72/Year
Efficacy	50% Risk reduction from meta-analysis
Cost Effective	Yes
Safety	Gastrointestinal bleed reduced by PPI use Intracranial bleed
Acceptable to Patients	Yes
Trial Phase	Case-control and cohort studies Phase III RCT in progress
Other Benefits	Cardioprotective

and NSAIDs 0.65 (95% CI, 0.46–0.92).[40] Farrow and colleagues[41] performed a population-based case-control study and found that patients who had used aspirin at least once per week for at least 6 months were associated with a decreased risk of EAC (OR, 0.37; 95% CI, 0.24–0.58), esophageal squamous carcinoma, and gastric adenocarcinoma. A similar relationship was seen with NSAIDs. An Irish case-control study looked at aspirin and NSAID use in patients with reflux esophagitis (230), BE (224), and EAC (227) and in controls (260). They found NSAID use lower in Barrett and EAC patients. The FINBAR study found patients who used aspirin showed a reduction in the relative risk of Barrett (OR 0.53; 95% CI, 0.31–0.9) and EAC (OR 0.57; 95% CI, 0.36–0.93). NSAID use had a reduced risk of BE (OR 0.4; 95% CI, 0.19–0.81) and EAC (OR 0.58; 0.31–1.08).[23] Patients with EAC and BE were less likely to use NSAIDs and aspirin. This result could be due to recall bias, exacerbation of reflux, or perception of Barrett being a contraindication or that it does exert a chemoprotective effect. The fact that aspirin and NSAIDs seem to reduce the risk of BE suggests the benefit may be exerted before Barrett forms. Cuziak and colleagues[9] presented data from two case-control and four cohort studies, finding a relative risk of developing esophageal cancer 0.41 (95% CI, 0.29–0.57) in the case-control studies and 0.83 (95% CI, 0.7–0.98) in the cohort studies of patients using aspirin. A pooled relative risk of 0.72 (95% CI, 0.62–0.84) was found when epidemiologic data, predominantly case-control studies, were reviewed.[42]

Aspirin is cost effective. An analysis of cost-effectiveness found aspirin as chemoprevention against Barrett adenocarcinoma cost effective, assuming a risk reduction of 50% and 0.5% per year progression rate.[43] Aspirin remained cost effective until risk reduction of 10% was assumed, indicating that even a small benefit is cost effective. Aspirin alone, or in combination with surveillance endoscopy, was cost effective. Aspirin is cheap, costing a few dollars per year.

Aspirin is acceptable to patients. Patient preference, essential in underpinning compliance, has been studied. Patients attending for Barrett surveillance endoscopies were questioned on their preferences on chemoprevention. As a group they were interested in the concept of chemoprevention. The investigators found 76% of patients were willing to take aspirin; the remaining patients were concerned about the risk of gastrointestinal bleeding. This was in contrast to 15% willing to take celecoxib to reduce future cancer risk, the remaining reluctant due the increased risk of myocardial infarction.[44] Aspirin could convey further protective benefits to patients with BE. A study of 245 deaths in a cohort of 1272 patients with BE found 21% died from cardiac disease. The cardioprotective benefits of aspirin in this group are a desirable effect.[29]

Negative issues regarding aspirin as a chemopreventative agent include emerging aspirin resistance. This has been reported in relation to failure to prevent ischemic episodes.[45] It is not known whether or not this would be a barrier to chemoprevention in some patients. Some large studies have shown no benefit in reducing cancer risk. The Physicians' Health Study, of 22,071 physicians randomized to aspirin (325 mg) or placebo, also found no benefit in taking aspirin for any cancer risk.[46] Nguyen and colleagues[26] performed a retrospective observational study on 344 patients with BE in an Veterans Affairs cohort with 2620 patient years of data. Aspirin and NSAID use was associated with a trend toward lower-risk HGD or EAC, but this did not reach statistical significance (HR 0.51; 95% CI, [0.25–1.04]). A retrospective analysis of the UK Barrett's Esophagus Registry found no significant difference in the HR of developing dysplasia or EAC in those taking aspirin over 3683 patient years of follow-up.[47]

An international consensus statement on aspirin and NSAIDs in chemoprevention has recently concluded that definitive recommendations cannot be made but that aspirin and sulindac had "very probable" antitumor effects.[9]

Minimizing Gastrointestinal Bleeds

The main drawback of using aspirin and NSAIDs as chemopreventive agents is the gastrointestinal side effects. They lead to gastropathy, resulting in dyspepsia, ulceration, upper gastrointestinal bleeding, and death.[48] This occurs via COX-1 inhibition. This risk increases with increasing age, as does the incidence of Barrett, peaking in the seventh decade. There is also an increased risk of hemorrhagic strokes, with 12 events per 10,000 patients in a meta-analysis of 16 trials with more than 55,000 patients.[49] A meta-analysis of 24 randomized control trials (RCTs), involving approximately 66,000 patients on 50 to1500 mg aspirin per day for a mean of 28 months, revealed a gastrointestinal hemorrhage in 2.47% of patients, compared with 1.42% of patients on placebo, with no apparent dose-dependent relationship.[50] Number needed to harm was 106 with 28 months' aspirin use (82–140) in the same analysis. All trials excluded high-risk patients with gastrointestinal bleed or ulceration, therefore perhaps these patients had a lower risk than the general population.[50] A multinational study of 187 patients on cardioprotective doses of aspirin found the prevalence of gastroduodenal ulcers at endoscopy was 11%, but the majority had no symptoms.[51] The OR of risk of gastrointestinal bleeding in aspirin as a cardioprotective agent has been reported at 1.5 to 3.1.[52] The incidence of gastrointestinal hemorrhage associated with aspirin is higher with increasing age. COX-2 inhibitors have fewer gastrointestinal side effects but enhanced cardiovascular risk, again, particularly in the elderly.

Methods used to reduce the risk of gastrointestinal hemorrhage associated with aspirin use include enteric-coated preparations, *Helicobacter pylori* eradication, and concomitant use of PPIs, histamine-2 receptor antagonists, and nitrous oxide (NO)-aspirin. Gastroprotective agents are used to reduce the risk of aspirin-induced gastrointestinal complications. Misoprostal (100 µg), a prostaglandin E analog, reduced the risk of erosions in a cohort of health volunteers on low-dose aspirin (OR 0.18),[53] but its use has been limited by the side-effect profile, in particular, diarrhea. Histamine-2 receptor antagonists reduce the risk of gastrointestinal bleeds in low-dose aspirin use; however, they are less effective than PPIs. A multicenter RCT compared 20 mg and 40 mg of omeprazole with ranitidine in ulcer healing, reduction in the number of erosions to less than 5, and symptomatic relief from dyspepsia. The found treatment success at 8 weeks in 80% of patients taking omeprazole (20 mg), 79% taking omeprazole (40 mg), and 63% of those taking ranitidine.[54] Enteric-coated preparations have not been found effective at reducing gastrointestinal complications. The risk of developing peptic ulceration in aspirin and NSAID use is increased by *Helicobacter pylori* infection. Eradication before starting these medications is associated with a lower risk of ulceration. A randomized trial of patients treated with diclofenac (100 mg) daily for 6 months was associated with a risk of 12.1% of developing an ulcer in the patients who underwent eradication, compared with 34.4% of the placebo group.[55]

The optimal dose of aspirin for cancer prevention is unknown. Findings from large population-based studies suggest that the dose may be higher than that needed to have a cardioprotective effect, thereby altering the risk-benefit ratio.[56] A combinatorial approach allows potentially lower doses of individual medications to be used, reducing adverse effects. Synergistic effects may result in addition multiple points of the metaplastic-dysplastic-adenocarcinoma spectrum could be targeted at the same time. An example of this synergistic combination could be PPIs and aspirin.[57]

AspECT

There are several recent and ongoing trials of chemoprevention in BE (**Table 2**). The Aspirin Esomeprazole Chemoprevention Trial (AspECT) is a phase III multicenter

Table 2
Chemoprevention trials for Barrett's esophagus

Trial	Primary Outcome Measures	Phase	Target/Number Enrolled	End Date
A Phase III, Randomized, Study of Aspirin and Esomeprazole Chemoprevention in Barrett's Metaplasia [ASPECT]	Conversion of BE to adenocarcinoma of the esophagus or HGD	Phase III	2513	2019
Randomized, Double-Blinded Phase II Trial of Esomeprazole Versus Esomeprazole + Two Doses of Aspirin in Barrett's Esophagus Patients	Change in mean tissue PGE2 concentration from the pre-intervention to the postintervention evaluation	Phase II	168	April 2009
Phase IIb Chemoprevention Trial of Difluoromethylornithine (DFMO) in Human Subjects With Intestinal-Type Barrett's Esophagus		Phase II completed	152	Completed
Clinical Studies on Bile Acids in Barrett's Esophagus	Protection against DNA damage by UDCA	Not stated	120	March 2014
Chemoprevention for Barrett's Esophagus Trial (CBET)	Determine the safety and efficacy of celecoxib for regression of Barrett dysplasia in patients with LGD or HGD of the esophagus	Phase II	100 Randomized	Published results
Phase IB Randomized, Double-Blinded, Placebo-Controlled, Dose Escalation Study of Polyphenon E in Patients With Barrett's Esophagus Green Tea Extract	Maximum tolerated dose of Poly E	Phase IB	40	December 2010

Effect of Antireflux Therapy on the Expression of Genes Known to be Important in Inflammation, Metaplasia and Neoplasia in Patients With GERD (Drug: Prevacid Solutabs Procedure: Antireflux surgery)	Gene expression Inflammation: IL-8, IFN-g, TNF-α, Intestinal metaplasia: CDX-1/2, MUC2 Neoplasia: COX-2, VEGF, and EGFR	Observational	40	December 2010
Clinical Study of Ursodeoxycholic Acid in Barrett's Patients With Low Grade Dysplasia	Reversal of oxidative DNA damage	Phase II	36	September 2012
Chemoprevention Trial Using Erlotinib in Barrett's Esophagus With High-Grade Dysplasia	Histologic regression of BE with HGD by chemoprevention with erlotinib hydrochloride	Phase I	25	Recruiting
A Pilot Study of the Effect of Sorafenib on Molecular Biomarkers in Barrett's Esophagus With High Grade Dysplasia	To characterize the effects of sorafenib on specific molecular markers in patients with BE and high-grade intraepithelial neoplasia or carcinoma in situ	Pilot study	15	May 2011
Pilot Study of Oral 852A for Elimination of High-Grade Dysplasia in Barrett's Esophagus	Elimination of HGD in Barrett's esophagus	Study terminated	10	October 2012

Abbreviations: CDX-1/2, caudal-type homeodomain transcription factors 1 and 2; IFN-g, interferon gamma; IL, interleukin; Poly E, polyphenon E; UDCA, ursodeoxycholic acid.

Data from Clinicaltrials.gov.

RCT. It is an open-label study with a 2 × 2 design. Patients were randomized to receive esomeprazole (80 mg or 20 mg) with or without low-dose aspirin (300 mg); 2513 patients have been recruited. The primary endpoints are all-cause mortality and reduction of HGD or EAC. Das and colleagues[58] report 85% to 90% of recruited patients remain on the initially randomized medications with no dose changes; 5% of patients have reduced or stopped aspirin and 3% have increased the esomeprazole dose to achieve symptomatic relief. The dropout rate from 2005 to 2009 was low, with 7% defaulting from further follow-up. AspECT is the largest RCT in BE and aims to address some of the major questions surrounding chemoprevention. Interim results are due in 2013. Since the introduction of AspECT, concordance with biopsy protocols has improved for all patients in centers recruiting patients even if individual patients were not taking part.[59]

TARGETING CHEMOPREVENTION

Risk of malignant transformation is limited to columnar-lined esophagus with the presence of specialized intestinal metaplasia (SIM). Risk of adenocarcinoma from BE in a Northern Ireland study showed cancer risk 0.26% per year for columnar-lined esophagus. This increased to 0.4% in the presence of specialized intestinal metaplasia and to more than 1% the subgroup of age 70 years and older with SIM.[60] The best current risk factor for developing EAC in BE is the presence of dysplasia. Although the general risk with Barrett is low, with an annual risk of 0.5% to 1% per annum, with LGD present the annual risk is 12%, rising to 14% to 28% when HGD is diagnosed. Esophagectomy studies have found 43% of patients undergoing esophagectomy for HGD had carcinoma in situ in their histology.[61] Macroscopic markers at endoscopy indicating high risk of advanced dysplasia or EAC, such as Barrett ulcer, nodule, stricture, or severe oesophagitis, led to 33.4 (95% CI, 3.8–289) increased risk of developing HGD or EAC compared with those who did not.[25] Based on evidence, patients with BE with SIM are at higher causes risk and should be targeted for chemoprevention. Those with visible lesions at endoscopy are also at higher risk and, therefore, should be targeted for chemoprevention. The development of knowledge regarding the role of biomarkers should help delineate those at most risk, thus allowing targeted chemoprevention in a more cost-effective manner. Patients with a high cardiovascular risk profile would also benefit from aspirin. Duration of treatment seems an unknown entity. Studies have suggested risk reduction commences at 10 years and increases with duration of chemoprevention. The most advantageous time to commence chemoprevention is proposed as 10 years before the peak onset of the cancer, the seventh decade for Barrett adenocarcinoma.

SUMMARY

A pill a day…? We are not quite there yet. There are currently no medications licensed for chemoprevention in BE; however, aspirin and other NSAIDs along with PPIs are promising agents. The largest RCT in the subject is currently taking place and the results, which are eagerly awaited, will help guide future practice.

REFERENCES

1. Falk GW, Jankowski J. Chemoprevention and Barrett's esophagus: decisions, decisions. Am J Gastroenterol 2008;103:2443–5.
2. Van Soest EM, Dieleman JP, Siersema PD, et al. Increasing incidence of Barrett's oesophagus in the general population. Gut 2005;54:1062–6.

3. Cameron AJ, Zinsmeister AR, Ballard DJ, et al. Prevalence of columnar-lined (Barrett's) esophagus. Comparison of population-based clinical and autopsy findings. Gastroenterology 1990;99:918–22.
4. Gatenby PA, Caygill CPJ, Ramus JR, et al. Barrett's columnar-lines oesophagus: demographic and lifestyle associations and adenocarcinoma risk. Dig Dis Sci 2008;53:1175–85.
5. Jankowski JA, Provenzale D, Moayyedi P. Esophageal adenocarcinoma arising from Barrett's metaplasia has regional variations in the West. Gastroenterology 2002;122:588–95.
6. Jankowska H, Hooper P, Jankowski JA. Aspirin chemoprevention of gastrointestinal cancer in the next decade. A review of the evidence. Pol Arch Med Wewn 2010;120(10):407–12.
7. Gatenby PA, Ramus JR, Caygill CP, et al. The Influence of symptom type and duration on the fate of the metaplastic columnar-lined oesophagus. Aliment Pharmacol Ther 2009;29:1096–105.
8. Skacel M, Petras RE, Gramlich TL, et al. The diagnosis of low-grade dysplasia in Barrett's esophagus and its implications for disease progression. Am J Gastroenterol 2000;95:3383–7.
9. Cuziak J, Otto F, Baron JA, et al. Aspirin and non-steroidal anti-inflammatory drugs for cancer prevention: an international consensus statement. Lancet Oncol 2009;10:501–7.
10. Sonnenberg A, Fennerty MB. Medical decision analysis of chemoprevention against esophageal adenocarcinoma. Gastroenterology 2003;124:1758–66.
11. Jankowski JA, Hawk ET. A methodologic analysis of chemoprevention and cancer prevention strategies for gastrointestinal cancer. Nat Clin Pract Gastroenterol Hepatol 2006;3:101–11.
12. Cook NR, Lee IM, Gaziano JM. Low-dose aspirin in the primary prevention of cancer. The women's health study: a randomized controlled trial. JAMA 2005; 294:47–55.
13. Freedman ND, Park Y, Subar AF, et al. Fruit and vegetable intake and esophageal cancer in a large prospective cohort study. Int J Cancer 2007;121:2753–60.
14. Chen H, Tucker KL, Graubard BI, et al. Nutrient intakes and adenocarcinoma of the esophagus and distal stomach. Nutr Cancer 2002;42:33–40.
15. Martin RC, Liu Q, Wo JM, et al. Chemoprevention of carcinogenic progression to esophageal adenocarcinoma by manganese superoxide dismutase supplementation. Clin Cancer Res 2007;13:176–82.
16. Lechpammer M, Xu X, Ellis HE Jr, et al. Flavopiridol reduces malignant transformation of the esophageal mucosa in p27 knockout mice. Oncogene 2005;24:1683–8.
17. Hormi-Carver K, Feagins LA, Spechler SJ, et al. All trans-retinoic acid induces apoptosis via p38 and caspase pathways in metaplastic Barrett's cells. Am J Physiol Gastrointest Liver Physiol 2007;292:G18–27.
18. Shammas MA, Koley H, Beer DG, et al. Growth arrest, apoptosis, and telomere shortening of Barrett's-associated adenocarcinoma cells by a telomerase inhibitor. Gastroenterology 2004;126:1337–46.
19. Kresty LA, Frankel WL, Hammond CD, et al. Transitioning from preclinical to clinical chemopreventive assessments of lyophilized black raspberries: interim results show berries modulate markers of oxidative stress in Barrett's esophagus patients. Nutr Cancer 2006;54:148–56.
20. Woodall CE, Li Y, Liu QH, et al. Chemoprevention of metaplasia initiation and cardiogenic progression to esophageal adenocarcinoma by resveratrol supplementation. Anticancer Drugs 2009;20:437–43.

21. Locke GR, Talley NJ, Fett SL, et al. Prevalence and clinical spectrum of gastro-esophageal reflux: a population-based study in Olmsted County, Minnesota. Gastroenterology 1997;112:1448–56.

22. Lagergren J, Bergstrom R, Lindgren A, et al. Symptomatic gastroesophageal reflux as a risk factor for esophageal adenocarcinoma. N Engl J Med 1999;340:825–31.

23. Anderson LA, Watson RG, Murphy SJ, et al. Risk factors for Barrett's oesophagus and oesophageal adenocarcinoma: results from the FINBAR study. World J Gastroenterol 2007;13:1585–94.

24. Ouatu-Lascar R, Triadafilopoulos G. Complete elimination of reflux symptoms does not guarantee normalisation of intraesophageal acid refluxing patients with Barrett's esophagus. Am J Gastroenterol 1998;93:711–6.

25. Hillman LC, Chiragakis L, Shadbolt B, et al. Proton-pump inhibitor therapy and the development of dysplasia in patients with Barrett's oesophagus. Med J Aust 2004;180:387–91.

26. Nguyen DM, El-Serag HB, Henderson L, et al. Medication usage and risk of neoplasia in patients with Barrett's esophagus. Clin Gastroenterol Hepatol 2009;7:1299–304.

27. Lao-Siriex P, Roy A, Worrall C, et al. Effect of acid suppression on molecular predictors for esophageal cancer. Cancer Epidemiol Biomarkers Prev 2006;15: 288–93.

28. Fitzgerald RC, Lascar R, Triadafilopoulos G. Barrett's oesophagus, dysplasia and pharmacologic acid suppression. Aliment Pharmacol Ther 2001;15:269–76.

29. Moayyedii P, Burch N, Akhtar-Danesh N, et al. Mortality rates in patients with Barrett's oesophagus. Aliment Pharmacol Ther 2008;27:316–20.

30. Mehta S, Boddy A, Johnson IT, et al. Systematic review: cyclo-oxygenase-2 in numan oesophageal adenocarcinogenesis. Aliment Pharmacol Ther 2006; 24:1321–31.

31. Buttar NS, Wang KK, Anderson MA, et al. Chemoprevention of esophageal adenocarcinoma by COX-2 inhibitors in an animal model of Barrett's esophagus. Gastroenterology 2002;122:1102–12.

32. Buttar NS, Wand KK, Anderson MA, et al. The effect of selective cyclooxygenase-2 inhibition in Barrett's esophagus epithelium: an in vitro study. J Natl Cancer Inst 2002;94:422–9.

33. Oyama K, Fujimara T, Ninomiya I, et al. A COX-2 inhibitor prevents the esophageal inflammation-metaplasia-adenocarcinoma sequence in rates. Carcinogenesis 2005;26:565–70.

34. Vaughan TL, Dong LM, Blount PL, et al. Non-steroidal anti-inflammatory drugs and risk of neoplastic progression in Barrett's oesophagus: a prospective study. Lancet Oncol 2005;6:945–52.

35. Heath EI, Canto MI, Paintadosi S. Secondary chemoprevention of Barrett's esophagus with celecoxib: results of a randomized trial. J Natl Cancer Inst 2007;99:545–57.

36. Shar AO, Guadard MA, Health EL, et al. Modelling using baseline characteristics in a small multicenter clinical trial for Barrett's esophagus. Contemp Clin Trials 2009;30:2–7.

37. Jacobson GA, Narkowicz C, Lord R, et al. Effect of celecoxib on cyclooxygenase-2 expression and possible variants in a patient with Barrett's esophagus. Dis Esophagus 2007;20:265–8.

38. Kaur BS, Khamnehel N, Iravani M, et al. Rofecoxib inhibits cyclooxygenase expression and activity and reduces cell proliferation in Barrett's esophagus. Gastroenterology 2002;123:60–7.

39. Corley DA, Kerlikowske K, Verma R, et al. Protective association of aspirin/NSAIDs and esophageal cancer: a systematic review and meta-analysis. Gastroenterology 2003;124:47–56.
40. Gonzalez-Perez A, Garcia Rodriguez LA, Lopez-Ridaura R. Effects of nonsteroidal anti-inflammatory drugs on cancer sites other than the colon and rectum: a meta-analysis. BMC Cancer 2003;3:28.
41. Farrow DC, Vaughan TL, Hansten PD, et al. Use of aspirin and other nonsteroidal anti-inflammatory drugs and risk of esophageal and gastric cancer. Cancer Epidemiol Biomarkers Prev 1998;7:97–102.
42. Bosetti C, Gallus S, Vecchia CL. Aspirin and cancer risk: an updated quantitative review to 2005. Cancer Causes Control 2006;17:871–88.
43. Hur C, Norman S, Nishioka G, et al. Cost-effectiveness of aspirin chemoprevention for Barrett's esophagus. J Natl Cancer Inst 2004;96:316–25.
44. Hur C, Broughton DE, Ozane E, et al. Patient preferences for the chemoprevention of esophageal adenocarcinoma in Barrett's esophagus. Am J Gastroenterol 2008;103:2432–42.
45. Hankey GJ, Eikelboom JW. Aspirin resistance. BMJ 2004;328:477–9.
46. Gann PH, Manson JE, Glynn RJ, et al. Low-dose aspirin and the incidence of colorectal tumors in a randomized trial. J Natl Cancer Inst 1993;85:1220–4.
47. Gatenby PA, Ramus JR, Caygill CP, et al. Aspirin is not chemoprotective for Barrett's adenocarcinoma of the oesophagus in a multicentre cohort. Eur J Cancer Prev 2009;18:381–4.
48. Goel A, Gasche C, Bolland R. Chemoprevention goes gourmet: different flavour of NO-aspirin. Mol Interv 2005;5:207–10.
49. He J, Whelton PK, Vu B, et al. Aspirin and risk of hemorrhagic stroke: a meta-analysis of randomized control trials. JAMA 1998;280:1930–5.
50. Derry S, Loke YK. Risk of gastrointestinal haemorrhage with long term use of aspirin: meta-analysis. BMJ 2000;321:1183–7.
51. Yeomans ND, Lanas AI, Talley NJ, et al. Prevalence and incidence of gastroduodenal ulcers during treatment with vascular protective doses of aspirin. Aliment Pharmacol Ther 2005;22:795–801.
52. Lanas A, Scheiman J. Low-dose aspirin and upper gastrointestinal damage: epidemiology, prevention and treatment. Curr Med Res Opin 2007;23:163–73.
53. Donelly MT, Goddard AF, Filipowicz B, et al. Low-dose misoprostol for the prevention of low-dose aspirin-induced gastroduodenal injury. Aliment Pharmacol Ther 2000;14:529–34.
54. Yeomans ND, Tulassay Z, Juhasz L, et al. A comparison of omeprazole with ranitidine for ulcers associated with nonsteroidal anti-inflammatory drugs. Acid suppression trial: ranitidine versus omeprazole for NSAID-associated ulcer treatment (ASTRONAUT) study group. N Engl J Med 1998;338:719–26.
55. Chan FK, To KF, Wu CJ, et al. Eradication of helicobacter pylori and risk of peptic ulcers in patients staring long term treatment with nonsteroidal anti-inflammatory drugs: a randomized trial. Lancet 2002;359:9–13.
56. Morgan G. Non-steroidal anti-inflammatory drugs and the chemoprevention of colorectal and oesophageal cancers. Gut 1996;38:646–8.
57. Dunn LJ, Jankowski J. Chemoprevention of gastrointestinal cancer. Br J Surg 2008;95:674–6.
58. Das D, Chilton AP, Jankowski JA. Chemoprevention of esophageal cancer and the AspECT trial. Recent Results Cancer Res 2009;181:161–8.

59. Das D, Ishaq S, Harrison R, et al. Management of Barrett's esophagus in the UK: overtreated and underbiopsied but improved by the introduction of a national randomized trial. Am J Gastroenterol 2008;103:1079–89.
60. Murray L, Watson P, Johnston B, et al. Risk of adenocarcinoma in Barrett's oesophagus: population based study. BMJ 2003;327:534–5.
61. Pellegrini CA, Pohl D. High-grade dysplasia in Barrett's esophagus: surveillance or operation. J Gastrointest Surg 2000;4:131–4.

Diagnosis and Management of Barrett's Esophagus: What's Next?

V. Raman Muthusamy, MD[a], Prateek Sharma, MD[b,c],*

KEYWORDS

- Barrett's esophagus • Future directions • Chemoprevention
- Screening • Surveillance • Endoscopic eradication

The past decade has led to marked improvements in the understanding regarding the pathogenesis and risk of progression of Barrett's esophagus (BE), enhanced imaging technology to improve dysplasia detection, and the development and refinement of endoscopic techniques, such as mucosal ablation and endoscopic mucosal resection, (EMR) to eradicate BE. However, many questions remain including identifying which, if any, candidates are most appropriate for screening for BE; how to improve current surveillance protocols; predicting which patients with BE will develop neoplastic progression; identifying the most appropriate candidates for endoscopic eradication therapy; developing algorithms for appropriate management posteradication; and understanding the potential role of chemoprophylaxis. This article describes potential future advances regarding screening, surveillance, risk stratification, endoscopic eradication therapies, and chemoprevention and provides a potential future management strategy for patients with BE.

SCREENING

Although conceptually attractive, screening for BE is complicated because of a variety of factors. At present, there is no clear evidence that screening reduces mortality rates due to esophageal adenocarcinoma. In addition, although BE is most common in elderly white men with chronic gastroesophageal reflux disease (GERD), only 40%

[a] Division of Gastroenterology, University of California, 101 The City Drive, City Tower, Suite 400, Zot 4092, Irvine, Orange, CA 92868, USA
[b] Division of Gastroenterology, Department of Medicine, University of Kansas Medical Center, Kansas City, KS, USA
[c] Division of Gastroenterology, Department of Medicine, Veterans Administration Medical Center, 4801 East Linwood Boulevard, Kansas City, MO 64128-2295, USA
* Corresponding author. Division of Gastroenterology, Department of Medicine, Veterans Affairs Medical Center, 4801 East Linwood Boulevard, Kansas City, MO 64128-2295.
E-mail address: psharma@kumc.edu

Gastrointest Endoscopy Clin N Am 21 (2011) 171–181
doi:10.1016/j.giec.2010.09.010
1052-5157/11/$ – see front matter. Published by Elsevier Inc.

of patients in some population-based studies of BE prevalence reported recent GERD symptoms.[1] Thus, screening using a history of recent GERD may miss over half of patients with BE. In addition, although obesity and dietary factors have been proposed as risk factors for the development of BE, there are currently no risk factors that reliably identify BE in asymptomatic patients. Furthermore, upper endoscopy, the current method of screening, is both costly and invasive. Given these difficulties, recent guidelines do not endorse population-based screening and only weakly recommend considering screening in elderly Caucasian men with frequent and long-standing GERD symptoms.[2]

In the future, screening may become feasible via the development of less invasive, inexpensive, and more accurate screening modalities. Recently, dedicated esophageal capsules (Pillcam ESO and PillcamESO2, Given Imaging, Yokneam, Israel) have been used as a minimally invasive technique to identify BE. The second generation of these devices nearly doubles the field of view, increases the depth of field, contains multiple lenses, and obtains up to 18 frames per second. Unfortunately, despite these improvements, this technique was found to have limited sensitivity for BE detection in several studies, while being less cost effective than esophagogastroduodenoscopy (EGD)-based screening.[3,4] Future advancements in capsule imaging, including single-fiber endoscopy using a tethered capsule with air insufflation capabilities, may make capsule-based BE screening a reality.[5,6] It is likely, however, that the most attractive future screening tool will not depend on direct visualization of the esophageal mucosa. Instead, it would detect BE via the examination of serum, saliva, or stool specimen for biomarkers that reliably predict the presence of BE. The development of a sensitive and inexpensive test using these easily obtained specimen could provide cost-effective, population-based screening. This test could consist of a single, or more likely multiple, biomarkers that would predict the presence of BE. An early version of such a device has been developed and consists of a capsule sponge that is ingested and removed via a string attached to the sponge. Using a biomarker, the trefoil factor 3 gene, which is expressed at high levels on the luminal surface of BE, but not in the normal esophagus or stomach, a sensitivity of 78% and a specificity of 94% was achieved for the detection of BE.[7] Using such a technique, those having a negative- or low-probability study would require no further evaluation, whereas those with a positive or high-probability test would undergo subsequent EGD to confirm the presence, length, and degree of dysplasia within the detected BE. A less optimal, but still useful, advance would be a similar test that could predict the likelihood of the development of BE in patients with clinical or endoscopic evidence of GERD.

SURVEILLANCE

At present, the frequency of endoscopic surveillance once BE has been detected is determined primarily by the highest grade of dysplasia present. In general, patients with newly diagnosed nondysplastic BE are recommended to have a repeat endoscopy in 1 year (primarily to detect dysplasia that may have been missed at the index endoscopy due to sampling error), followed by further surveillance endoscopies every 3 years. Patients with low-grade dysplasia (LGD) typically have a repeat endoscopy every 6 months, whereas patients with high-grade dysplasia (HGD) not electing immediate endoscopic or surgical therapy undergo surveillance biopsies at 3-month intervals. Although surveillance does seem to lead to increased detection of early-stage esophageal adenocarcinoma, clear evidence that this practice leads to a disease-specific mortality reduction is lacking.[8,9] Furthermore, endoscopists frequently do not follow the recommended protocol, with one study showing an overall compliance rate of 51.2% in the United States.[10] Similarly, poor adherence rates were also seen in the Netherlands, with worsening compliance with increasing length of Barrett's epithelium seen in both countries.[10,11] In addition, even if performed appropriately, only 4% to 6% of the metaplastic region is sampled, and routine surveillance of all patients with BE incurs considerable expense and inconvenience. Given these limitations, several enhancements to our current practice of endoscopic surveillance are desired.

First among these is the development of systematic reporting and the performance of a careful, standardized Barrett withdrawal technique, similar to what is currently emphasized for colonoscopy. Routine documentation of key esophageal landmarks, washing of the esophageal epithelium, usage of validated BE measuring systems (Prague Criteria), performance of a careful visual examination of the esophagus using advanced imaging technologies, and adherence to biopsy technique and protocols should be expected and used as an endoscopic quality metric. The use of his quality metric will hopefully improve dysplasia detection and reduce the need for repeat surveillance biopsies in patients being considered for endoscopic eradication therapies due to poor documentation or biopsy protocol. In addition, multicenter trials are needed to prospectively assess the impact of surveillance on disease-specific survival. Last, risk stratification to determine who would benefit most from this approach is arguably the most important future advance regarding surveillance and would markedly improve the cost effectiveness of this approach.

In addition to enhancements in the process of surveillance, several endoscopic imaging advancements have been made to improve the efficiency and diagnostic yield of surveillance biopsies in detecting dysplasia or early neoplasia. These advancements have included high-definition imaging, image magnification, and narrow band imaging (NBI) that are built in to many current endoscopes. In addition, technologies such as autofluorescence imaging and confocal laser endomicroscopy (CLE) have also been used to enhance dysplasia detection and to provide "real-time" histology, leading to the ability to provide immediate therapy via EMR. In the near future, surveillance protocols could be altered to incorporate many of these technologies. For example, it seems that NBI combined with high-definition white-light endoscopy may increase the detection of dysplastic lesions with a reduction in the number of needed biopsies.[12,13] For the vast majority of patients without dysplasia, future surveillance could involve having the entire BE region being assessed with NBI/high-definition white light endoscopy, and if no high-risk lesions are seen, random 4-quadrant probe-based CLE could be performed in a fashion similar to obtaining biopsies. For patients without visualized abnormalities on CLE, biopsies could be avoided altogether, whereas those with abnormalities on either white-light, NBI, or probe-based CLE would undergo targeted biopsies of the identified potentially dysplastic regions in addition to random 4-quadrant biopsies every 2 cm. Such a strategy has the potential to reduce the number of biopsies taken in low-risk surveillance of nondysplastic BE by 10 fold, with about 2 of 3 of patients requiring no biopsies.[14]

On the more distant horizon, techniques using in-vivo molecular imaging such as fluorescence endoscopy using proflavine or indocyanine green may supplant video endoscopy as the preferred method used to initially scan the entire region of BE for dysplasia. These methods may be used to detect highly sensitive and specific whole or partial antibodies, nanoparticles, or peptide markers of dysplasia/malignancy within the BE segment.[15] These identified regions could then be marked and immediately interrogated via probe-based CLE and, if confirmed to contain abnormal tissue, undergo immediate EMR. This EMR would allow for a rapid, highly accurate method for immediate eradication of dysplasia/early cancer while avoiding the need for random biopsies altogether. Further advances in CLE are also anticipated, including multiphoton CLE that would avoid the need for an injected contrast agent (fluoroscein) by using autofluorescence from endogenous flavins and collagen. This device could provide subcellular imaging while adding information regarding biochemical/metabolic activity to the cellular imaging and structural data obtained by current single photon CLE devices. It is hoped that by using a combination of these approaches, a more limited, economical, and effective surveillance system can be developed and used in those most likely to benefit from close observation.

RISK STRATIFICATION

Of all the potential advances regarding BE, the ability to accurately risk stratify patients into categories according to their potential for neoplastic progression would seem to be the most significant. Currently, the primary method of stratification is based on the grade of dysplasia detected by endoscopic biopsies, and this information is used to set the recommended intervals for endoscopic surveillance. However, the grade of dysplasia detected may be subject to sampling error, and other important but currently ill-defined, clinical, and biochemical factors may more accurately predict the risk of progression to cancer. Thus, the concept of a composite panel that incorporates these clinical and biochemical risk factors with the current dysplasia-grade approach and can be easily obtained, possibly by nonendoscopic methods, and compiled into a Barrett Risk Score is very attractive. It has the potential to function similar to the Model for End-Stage Liver Disease Score for predicting liver failure in those with hepatic dysfunction. Before this risk score is achieved, however, much work is needed to identify which factors or biomarkers are significant and the magnitude of the risk of progression they confer.

A variety of patient predictors have been proposed including age, gender, body mass index/abdominal obesity, tobacco use, and diets with high fat and low fruit or vegetable intake. Despite some data suggesting that gender and dietary habits may truly be risk factors for BE progression to dysplasia, there is insufficient data at present to clearly identify any of these as clear risk factors. Furthermore, some factors such as gender and abdominal obesity are related, and so it remains unclear if these are truly independent criteria. In addition to these patient characteristics, other predictive criteria from endoscopic and histologic evaluation have been proposed, including BE length, nodularity at endoscopy, hiatal hernia size, and the grade and extent of dysplasia present. Similar to the proposed patient factors, several of these variables are subject to confounding, such as increasing BE length being associated with a higher prevalence of dysplasia. The independence and significance of these clinical variables await validation through large-scale prospective multi-center trials.

Many have proposed biomarkers as the ultimate indicators that will predict the potential for the development of HGD or cancer in a segment of BE. A variety of biomarkers have been proposed to date using the metaplasia-dysplasia-adenocarcinoma sequence in BE.[16] One class includes oncogenes that lead to uncontrolled cell proliferation such as cyclin D1, cyclin E, transforming growth factor α, epidermal growth factor, and epidermal growth factor receptor.[17] A second group of biomarkers inactivate tumor suppressor genes and lead to uncontrolled cell proliferation. Candidate genes include p16, p53, and the adenomatous polyposis mutation. Inactivation can occur by mutation, deletion of the chromosomal region encoding the gene (called loss of heterozygosity [LOH]), or the attachment of methyl groups to the promoter region of these genes leading to gene inactivation. Other proposed biomarker abnormalities result in the ability to avoid apoptosis (cyclooxygenase [COX]) 2 upregulation, Fas-ligand expression), undergo unlimited cell replication (telomerase expression), sustain angiogenesis (increased vascular endothelial growth factor and receptor expression), and invade and metastasize (E-cadherin, B-catenin expression). To date, the biomarkers that have shown the most promise in predicting neoplastic progression in BE are aneuploidy and increased tetraploidy (alterations in the normal diploid/tetraploid DNA content of cells), and LOH for p53 and p16.[18]

However, the identification and validation of biomarkers to predict progression to cancer is a complex and laborious process. Six phases have been proposed in biomarker development.[19,20] These distinct phases aim to identify (1) potential biomarkers via known or suspected models of neoplastic progression; (2) the ability of the proposed biomarker to distinguish between subjects with and without dysplasia/cancer via cross-sectional studies; (3) the ability of the biomarker to detect disease before its clinical diagnosis via case-control studies; (4) the extent and characteristics of the disease that is detected by the biomarker assay when used prospectively; (5) the ability of the test to reduce disease burden on the population; and (6) the demonstration of this ability) across multiple sites. At present, little data on biomarkers have been achieved beyond phase 3, and no phase 5 data are available. Data from large prospective studies such as the Aspirin Esomeprazole Chemoprevention Trial (AspECT) Chemoprevention Trial[21] (discussed later in this article) may provide tissue to achieve phase 4, but these would still need to be tested in a phase 5 trial, which would require many years. Thus, the creation and validation of such biomarker panels will require considerable time, effort, and expense. As a result, accurate biomarker panels will likely not be available for several years.

In addition to the time needed to develop and validate biomarker panels, several other issues present challenges to creating risk scores that incorporate biomarker panels. First, obtaining and storing the tissue used to obtain biomarkers is currently problematic, and streamlining the process of tissue acquisition and preservation before biomarker analysis are needed. Second, the methods for testing for these biomarkers such as fluorescence in situ hybridization and flow cytometry will require simplification and broader availability before they can be used in widespread clinical practice. Finally, and most significant, biomarker testing relies on the assumption that molecular abnormalities identified arise from 1 dominant clone. However, BE has shown multiple independent clones (polyclonality), suggesting that many different crypts that may not contribute to the overall molecular profile of the tissue sample may display dysplastic potential.[22] This display of dysplastic potential will lead to significant issues regarding biomarker panel validation and may require inclusion of several biomarkers in a panel to accurately predict the potential for neoplastic progression.

Despite these obstacles, once created and validated, a Barrett Risk Score could be used to divide patients into distinct risk groups. One possible model would be to stratify patients into 3 categories: those at very low risk, those at low-intermediate risk, and those at high risk for neoplastic progression. Those with a very low risk, who would likely comprise the vast majority of patients with nondysplastic BE and even some patients with LGD, could potentially avoid any further surveillance. Those at low-intermediate risk would undergo surveillance using the advanced imaging techniques previously described and also be potentially treated with chemopreventive agents to reduce their risk of progression and avoid the need for future endoscopic or surgical therapy. Those at high risk, who would likely be comprised of those patients with HGD as well as select LGD and nondysplastic patients with BE, would undergo immediate treatment with endoscopic eradication techniques. Such an approach would limit eradication therapy to those most benefiting from treatment, while avoiding the cost, anxiety, and inconvenience of surveillance in the majority of patients with BE.

ENDOSCOPIC THERAPY

Over the past 15 years, a variety of endoscopic eradication techniques for BE have been developed. These include techniques in which the tissue is ablated or resected and retrieved (EMR). Ablation can be achieved via a variety of mechanisms including thermal techniques, rapid mucosal cooling (cryotherapy), or using a photochemical reaction (photodynamic therapy) to achieve tissue destruction. Thermal ablation therapy initially used laser therapy, multipolar electrocoagulation, or argon plasma coagulation but more recently has evolved to the use of radiofrequency (RF) energy. As these techniques have been refined and data regarding their use have been accumulated, they have increasingly gained acceptance as an alternative to surgery in the treatment of patients with HGD. At present, given persistent uncertainty regarding the durability and cost effectiveness of these techniques, most societies recommend limiting the use of these therapies to patients with HGD, where the risk of progression to cancer is the greatest. Current recommendations are that nodular disease be removed via EMR to exclude invasive cancer and achieve mucosal eradication, with residual flat BE undergoing ablation, typically using RF energy.

In the future, the authors anticipate several additional advancements in endoscopic eradication technologies. These could include new techniques and equipment to perform wide-field, rapid, and safe endoscopic submucosal dissection that would allow for nonpiecemeal resection of large regions of BE. In addition, the concept of a single ablation modality that could be adjusted to treat varying lengths of BE, such as an incrementally inflatable balloon, while achieving a variety of ablation depths based on the amount of energy selected to be delivered is very appealing and would help to streamline the current array of ablative options. Once ablation is achieved, more data are also needed regarding the nature and durability of the neosquamous epithelium. In particular, endoscopic ablation becomes particularly attractive from an economic perspective if long-term durability of the neosquamous epithelium can be demonstrated after ablation, allowing for the discontinuation of routine postablation endoscopic surveillance. Another important issue is the frequency and long-term significance of subsquamous BE present under the postablation neosquamous epithelium. Given the concern that mucosal biopsies frequently do not achieve a depth sufficient to examine the lamina propria, how will such areas be identified? One potential technique is 3-dimensional optical coherence tomography, which combines high-resolution imaging, a large field of view, and rapid data acquisition.[23] This technique allows for broad subsurface assessment of patients who have undergone endoscopic ablation therapy and can identify isolated glands buried between 300 to 500 μm of neosquamous epithelium and lamina propria. Although the use of CLE currently for such a purpose is technically impractical and cumbersome, future advances in CLE may allow for a similar capability to detect subsquamous glandular mucosa over a broad region. These remaining uncertainties regarding endoscopic eradication techniques, coupled with the very low rates of neoplastic progression seen in LGD and nondysplastic BE, make it seem very unlikely that routine ablation of all patients with either of these histologic grades will ever become standard practice, especially if valid risk-stratification strategies can be developed.

In addition to the key questions regarding who should receive endoscopic eradication therapy and the duration and mechanism of the postsurveillance follow-up, several additional key questions remain regarding the choice of endoscopic therapy.

To start, can circumferential EMR of short regions be performed without significant stricturing? If so, for patients with short-segment BE, is EMR preferable to ablation therapy given that it allows for evaluation of the resected specimen to document complete BE removal? In addition, are there differences in the durability of the neosquamous epithelium obtained from resection and ablation techniques? Finally, are there specific advantages of one ablation technique compared with others that would lead to preferential of use of a specific modality in patients with certain anatomic, endoscopic, or histologic criteria? The authors anticipate that the next decade will provide many answers regarding technique optimization, efficacy, durability, and safety that are essential for continued and more widespread adoption of these modalities.

CHEMOPREVENTION

Chemoprevention, defined as a pharmacologic intervention that either prevents cancer or treats identified precancerous lesions,[24] is an attractive concept for patients with BE aiming to avoid the development of HGD or esophageal adenocarcinoma. At present, however, no clearly effective chemotherapeutic agents have been identified, and the use of proposed agents in current clinical practice is not recommended.[2] Two potential methods of chemoprophylaxis exist: primary and secondary. In primary chemoprophylaxis, a chemoprophylactic agent is administered broadly to the general population, rather than being limited to those with known precancerous lesions. This approach seems to have limited utility regarding BE and esophageal adenocarcinoma because only a small fraction of the population has BE, and vast majority of these patients will never develop dysplasia or cancer. Thus, subjecting the general population to the long-term expense and potential complications of the chemoprophylactic agents would seem to be ill advised, given the small number of patients who would potentially benefit from such treatment. Even the concept of treating a high-risk subset of the general population seems unfeasible, given the fact that the majority of patients with BE may lack characteristic clinical symptoms such as reflux.[1] Secondary prophylaxis, which is more limited in nature, is offered as treatment only to patients with identified precancerous lesions such as BE. This, unlike primary prophylaxis, seems to be a reasonable option in BE, particularly for those with at least some potential for malignant transformation. The concept of risk stratification is again attractive here, as secondary chemoprophylaxis would seem best reserved for those with some identified risk factors for neoplastic progression based on a clinical and/or biomarker-based risk panel. This concept would avoid the long-term expense, inconvenience, and risk of medication side effects that would result from treating the vast majority of patients with BE who are at very low risk to ever exhibit dysplastic progression.

   Several classes of medications have been proposed as chemoprophylactic agents. To date, proton-pump inhibitors (PPIs), aspirin (ASA), nonsteroidal anti-inflammatory agents (NSAIDS), and COX-2 inhibitors have been the most studied agents in BE. Other proposed agents include difluoromethylornithine and statin medications. Acid suppression is believed to potentially reduce neoplastic progression by reducing inflammation and markers of proliferation in BE,[25] although there is concern that acid suppression may lead to a predominantly bilious refluxate that could actually promote neoplastic change.[26] COX-2 overexpression has been detected in BE, and in-vitro studies suggest it promotes angiogenesis, increases the invasive nature of malignant cells, and reduces apoptosis rates.[27] Selective (COX-2) and nonselective (ASA, NSAIDS) inhibitors of COX-2 production are believed to counteract these mechanisms and thereby reduce neoplastic progression.[28] Although retrospective data and epidemiologic studies have shown a benefit of ASA and NSAIDS in reducing the progression to cancer in patients with BE,[29] a prospective trial of chemoprevention trial assessing a COX-2 inhibitor, celecoxib (200 mg twice daily for 48 weeks), failed to show a reduction in progression of patients with dysplasia to cancer.[30] Given that many patients with BE require PPI therapy to maintain healing of esophagitis or control reflux symptoms, use NSAIDs to treat arthritic pain, and may need ASA for its effects on inhibiting platelet activity, these agents are particularly attractive as chemoprevention agents as many patients with BE may require their use anyways.

These agents, however, are also associated with numerous side effects that should be considered before their use for a primarily chemopreventive indication. ASA increases the risk of gastrointestinal and cerebrovascular bleeding, NSAIDS can cause gastrointestinal distress/bleeding and renal dysfunction, and COX-2 inhibitors have been associated with an increase in myocardial infarctions. In addition, PPI therapy may affect absorption of calcium and certain medications, increase the risk of hip fractures, and increase the risk of pulmonary, foodborne, and *Clostridium dificile* infections.[31,32] Thus, any potential benefits from these agents regarding chemoprevention must be weighed against their potential side effects and complications. This is particularly important in BE, where the progression to cancer and cancer-specific mortality is extremely low. Fortunately, some important data regarding these agents should be coming shortly with the analysis of a large randomized European study (AspECT) of several thousand patients with BE assessing the role of low- or high-dose PPI with or without low-dose aspirin (300 mg) in reducing the risk of progression to cancer.[21]

Although the most data regarding chemoprevention have focused on pharmacologic therapy, the ideal candidate agent would be inexpensive, easily available, effective, safe, result in minimal to no side effects, and be naturally available. Thus, in addition to pharmaceuticals, several dietary chemopreventive factors have been proposed.[28,33] Antioxidants such as vitamin C, E, and carotenoids have been proposed to bind with reactive oxygen species produced from inflammation due to chronic acid and bile reflux. Similarly, diets high in fruit and vegetable intake, berry consumption, or green tea intake have been advocated because of their being enriched with antioxidants. To date, however, limited and often conflicting data exist regarding these agents in the prevention of BE or esophageal adenocarcinoma. Thus, despite the attractiveness of these agents from a cost and availability standpoint, future prospective and randomized trials are needed to further assess and validate the promise of these theories.

SUMMARY

The past decade has seen marked advances in the understanding of the risk of neoplastic progression in BE and the development of numerous modalities to achieve endoscopic eradication of this tissue. The next decade will hopefully yield numerous additional breakthroughs including identifying candidates appropriate for endoscopic screening or the development of inexpensive and noninvasive screening tests for the general population, imaging advances that improve dysplasia detection during surveillance, the development of clinical and biomarker panels for accurate risk stratification, the identification of effective chemoprophylactic agents, and an improved understanding of the most appropriate endoscopic eradication technique for a given clinical situation. A proposed algorithm of how potential advances in these areas could affect future management of patients with BE is shown in **Fig. 1**. Such an approach would improve BE detection, reduce the expense and patient anxiety associated with surveillance in patients with minimal risk of progression, and allow eradication

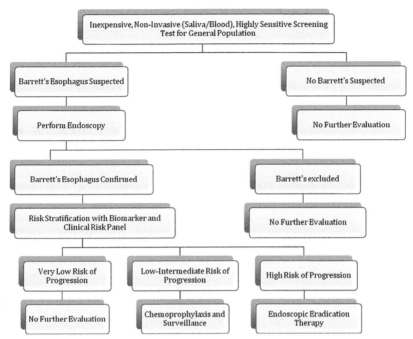

Fig. 1. Proposed future evaluation algorithm for BE.

techniques to be targeted to those most likely to benefit from their use. With continued progress, a reversal in the decades old rise in the incidence of and mortality from esophageal adenocarcinoma appears attainable.

REFERENCES

1. Ronkainen J, Aro P, Storskrubb T, et al. Prevalence of Barrett's esophagus in the general population: an endoscopic study. Gastroenterology 2005;129:1825–31.
2. Wang KK, Sampliner RE. Updated guidelines 2008 for the diagnosis, surveillance and therapy of Barrett's esophagus. Am J Gastroenterol 2008;103:788–97.
3. Waterman M, Gralnek IM. Capsule endoscopy of the esophagus. J Clin Gastroenterol 2009;43:605–12.
4. Bhardwaj A, Hollenbeak CS, Pooran N, et al. A meta-analysis of the diagnostic accuracy of esophageal capsule endoscopy for Barrett's esophagus in patients with gastroesophageal reflux disease. Am J Gastroenterol 2009;104:1533–9.
5. Seibel EJ, Carroll RE, Dominitz JA, et al. Tethered capsule endoscopy, a low-cost and high-performance alternative technology for the screening of esophageal cancer and Barrett's esophagus. IEEE Trans Biomed Eng 2008;55:1032–42.
6. Seibel EJ, Brown CM, Dominitz JA, et al. Scanning single fiber endoscopy: a new platform technology for integrated laser imaging, diagnosis, and future therapies. Gastrointest Endosc Clin N Am 2008;18:467–78, viii.
7. Lao-Sirieix P, Boussioutas A, Kadri SR, et al. Non-endoscopic screening biomarkers for Barrett's oesophagus: from microarray analysis to the clinic. Gut 2009;58:1451–9.
8. Cooper GS, Kou TD, Chak A. Receipt of previous diagnoses and endoscopy and outcome from esophageal adenocarcinoma: a population-based study with temporal trends. Am J Gastroenterol 2009;104:1356–62.

9. Corley DA, Levin TR, Habel LA, et al. Surveillance and survival in Barrett's adeno-carcinomas: a population-based study. Gastroenterology 2002;122:633–40.

10. Abrams JA, Kapel RC, Lindberg GM, et al. Adherence to biopsy guidelines for Barrett's esophagus surveillance in the community setting in the United States. Clin Gastroenterol Hepatol 2009;7:736–42 [quiz: 710].

11. Curvers WL, Peters FP, Elzer B, et al. Quality of Barrett's surveillance in The Netherlands: a standardized review of endoscopy and pathology reports. Eur J Gastroenterol Hepatol 2008;20:601–7.

12. Wolfsen HC, Crook JE, Krishna M, et al. Prospective, controlled tandem endoscopy study of narrow band imaging for dysplasia detection in Barrett's Esophagus. Gastroenterology 2008;135:24–31.

13. Sharma P, Bansal A, Mathur S, et al. The utility of a novel narrow band imaging endoscopy system in patients with Barrett's esophagus. Gastrointest Endosc 2006;64:167–75.

14. Dunbar KB, Okolo P 3rd, Montgomery E, et al. Confocal laser endomicroscopy in Barrett's esophagus and endoscopically inapparent Barrett's neoplasia: a prospective, randomized, double-blind, controlled, crossover trial. Gastrointest Endosc 2009;70:645–54.

15. Hsiung PL, Hardy J, Friedland S, et al. Detection of colonic dysplasia in vivo using a targeted heptapeptide and confocal microendoscopy. Nat Med 2008;14:454–8.

16. Nicholson A, Jankowski J. Editorial: One small step for metaplasia, but one giant leap for biomarkers is needed. Am J Gastroenterol 2009;104:2681–3.

17. Souza R. The molecular basis of carcinogenesis in Barrett's esophagus. J Gastrointest Surg 2010;14:937–40.

18. Prasad GA, Bansal A, Sharma P, et al. Predictors of progression in Barrett's esophagus: current knowledge and future directions. Am J Gastroenterol 2010; 105:1490–502.

19. Pepe MS, Etzioni R, Feng Z, et al. Phases of biomarker development for early detection of cancer. J Natl Cancer Inst 2001;93:1054–61.

20. Jankowski JA, Odze RD. Biomarkers in gastroenterology: between hope and hype comes histopathology. Am J Gastroenterol 2009;104:1093–6.

21. Das D, Ishaq S, Harrison R, et al. Management of Barrett's esophagus in the UK: overtreated and underbiopsied but improved by the introduction of a national randomized trial. Am J Gastroenterol 2008;103:1079–89.

22. Leedham SJ, Preston SL, McDonald SA, et al. Individual crypt genetic heterogeneity and the origin of metaplastic glandular epithelium in human Barrett's oesophagus. Gut 2008;57:1041–8.

23. Adler DC, Zhou C, Tsai TH, et al. Three-dimensional optical coherence tomography of Barrett's esophagus and buried glands beneath neosquamous epithelium following radiofrequency ablation. Endoscopy 2009;41:773–6.

24. Kelloff GJ, Lippman SM, Dannenberg AJ, et al. Progress in chemoprevention drug development: the promise of molecular biomarkers for prevention of intraepithelial neoplasia and cancer–a plan to move forward. Clin Cancer Res 2006;12:3661–97.

25. Leedham S, Jankowski J. The evidence base of proton pump inhibitor chemopreventative agents in Barrett's esophagus–the good, the bad, and the flawed! Am J Gastroenterol 2007;102:21–3.

26. Kaur BS, Ouatu-Lascar R, Omary MB, et al. Bile salts induce or blunt cell proliferation in Barrett's esophagus in an acid-dependent fashion. Am J Physiol Gastrointest Liver Physiol 2000;278:G1000–9.

27. Wilson KT, Fu S, Ramanujam KS, et al. Increased expression of inducible nitric oxide synthase and cyclooxygenase-2 in Barrett's esophagus and associated adenocarcinomas. Cancer Res 1998;58:2929–34.

28. Neumann H, Monkemuller K, Vieth M, et al. Chemoprevention of adenocarcinoma associated with Barrett's esophagus: potential options. Dig Dis 2009;27:18–23.
29. Corley DA, Kerlikowske K, Verma R, et al. Protective association of aspirin/ NSAIDs and esophageal cancer: a systematic review and meta-analysis. Gastroenterology 2003;124:47–56.
30. Heath EI, Canto MI, Piantadosi S, et al. Secondary chemoprevention of Barrett's esophagus with celecoxib: results of a randomized trial. J Natl Cancer Inst 2007; 99:545–57.
31. Corley DA, Kubo A, Zhao W, et al. Proton pump inhibitors and histamine-2 receptor antagonists are associated with hip fractures among at-risk patients. Gastroenterology 2010;139:93–101.
32. Corley DA. Chemoprevention in Barrett's esophagus: are we there yet, are we there yet? Clin Gastroenterol Hepatol 2009;7:1266–8.
33. Kubo A, Corley DA, Jensen CD, et al. Dietary factors and the risks of oesophageal adenocarcinoma and Barrett's oesophagus. Nutr Res Rev 2010;1–17.

Index

Note: Page numbers of article titles are in **boldface** type.

A

Ablation, radiofrequency. See *Radiofrequency ablation (RFA)*.
Adenocarcinoma
    early, in Barrett's esophagus, staging of, **53–66**. See also *Barrett's esophagus, early adenocarcinoma in, staging of.*
    esophageal. See *Esophageal adenocarcinoma.*
    HGD and, 140–141
5-ALA. See *5-Aminolevulinic acid (5-ALA).*
5-Aminolevulinic acid (5-ALA), PDT with, for Barrett's esophagus, 73–74
Anti-inflammatory drugs, nonsteroidal, in chemoprevention of Barrett's esophagus,
    160–162
Antioxidants, in chemoprevention of Barrett's esophagus, 158
AspECT, in chemoprevention of Barrett's esophagus, 163–166
Aspirin, in chemoprevention of Barrett's esophagus, 160–162

B

Barrett metaplasia
    CDX1 in, 28
    CDX2 in, 28
    GERD and, 28–30
    making of, 26
    management of, 139
    SOX9 in, 28
    through stem cells, 26–28
    transdifferentiation in, 26
Barrett-associated dysplasia, making of, esophageal adenocarcinoma and, 30
Barrett's esophagus, **1–7**
    biology of, **25–38**
        described, 25–26
    cancer risk associated with, 3–4
    chemoprevention in, **155–170**, 177–178
        agents in, 157–160
            antioxidants, 158
            aspirin, 160–162
            cyclin-dependent kinase inhibitors, 158
            food groups, 157–158
            lyophilized black raspberries, 159
            NSAIDs, 160–162
            polyphenols, 159
            proton pump inhibitors, 159–160
            retinoic acid, 159

Gastrointest Endoscopy Clin N Am 21 (2011) 183–188
doi:10.1016/S1052-5157(10)00144-3
1052-5157/11/$ – see front matter © 2011 Elsevier Inc. All rights reserved.

giendo.theclinics.com

Moving?

Make sure your subscription moves with you!

To notify us of your new address, find your **Clinics Account Number** (located on your mailing label above your name), and contact customer service at:

Email: **journalscustomerservice-usa@elsevier.com**

800-654-2452 (subscribers in the U.S. & Canada)
314-447-8871 (subscribers outside of the U.S. & Canada)

Fax number: 314-447-8029

Elsevier Health Sciences Division
Subscription Customer Service
3251 Riverport Lane
Maryland Heights, MO 63043

*To ensure uninterrupted delivery of your subscription, please notify us at least 4 weeks in advance of move.

ELSEVIER

Printed and bound by CPI Group (UK) Ltd, Croydon, CR0 4YY

03/10/2024

01040455-0018